TABLE OF CONTENTS

Top 20 Test Taking Tips

1. Carefully follow all the test registration procedures
2. Know the test directions, duration, topics, question types, how many questions
3. Setup a flexible study schedule at least 3-4 weeks before test day
4. Study during the time of day you are most alert, relaxed, and stress free
5. Maximize your learning style; visual learner use visual study aids, auditory learner use auditory study aids
6. Focus on your weakest knowledge base
7. Find a study partner to review with and help clarify questions
8. Practice, practice, practice
9. Get a good night's sleep; don't try to cram the night before the test
10. Eat a well balanced meal
11. Know the exact physical location of the testing site; drive the route to the site prior to test day
12. Bring a set of ear plugs; the testing center could be noisy
13. Wear comfortable, loose fitting, layered clothing to the testing center; prepare for it to be either cold or hot during the test
14. Bring at least 2 current forms of ID to the testing center
15. Arrive to the test early; be prepared to wait and be patient
16. Eliminate the obviously wrong answer choices, then guess the first remaining choice
17. Pace yourself; don't rush, but keep working and move on if you get stuck
18. Maintain a positive attitude even if the test is going poorly
19. Keep your first answer unless you are positive it is wrong
20. Check your work, don't make a careless mistake

Facilitate Learning

Education and nursing processes

The education process is an organized, well-planned course of action that correlates two major operations dependent on one another, teaching and learning. Together, the teacher and the student perform teaching and learning tasks to reach a desired goal of behavioral change. The changes that take place should create both student and teacher growth. The process should be participatory in nature, and should incorporate a mutual approach to both teaching and learning. It is appropriate to compare the education process with the nursing process, as both processes include the basic elements of assessment, planning, implementation, and evaluation.

The basic steps of the education process and the nursing process should correlate. Both processes provide a logical foundation for nursing practice. Both should include the fundamental steps of assessment, planning, implementation, and evaluation. These processes are ongoing with the need to take the results of assessment and evaluation, and redirect or refine planning and implementation.

The education and nursing processes differ in the focus of the planning and implementation phases. The education process must take into consideration the prioritization and assessment of the client's learning needs, style of learning, and preparedness to learn. The nursing process must focus on the patient's physical and psychosocial needs. Different outcomes are expected from both processes. The education process outcome is achieved when there is an alteration in knowledge, skill, and attitude in the student. The nursing process outcome is achieved when the client's physical and psychosocial needs are met. If outcomes are not achieved in either process, then the processes should begin again after reassessment, redesigning, and reimplementation.

Ability to learn

Several factors may affect an adult's ability to learn, among them the possibility that some adults never reach Jean Piaget's formal operations stage of development, meaning these adults will require a more concrete style of learning. A person who lacks an education may also demonstrate lower stages of thinking. The lower stages of thinking in adults may also be linked to disease, extraordinary stress, adverse effects of medication, and depression. Other factors that may interfere with adult learning include the demands of everyday life and personal childhood experiences. Adults may also have different perceptions of the presented information due to societal influences. These influences include cultural background, gender, ethnicity, social class, and their own self-concept.

Teaching strategies based student background

If the student is assessed as being in the formal operations stage, various teaching strategies can be utilized. Assess the students' motivation to learn, based on their background and assessed needs. Draw on the students' meaningful experiences with relationship to their background. Encourage them to set their own learning pace or be self-directed. Computer-assisted instruction can be effectively incorporated. Role playing or hands-on practice can be utilized. Provide information which will coincide with the students' own concerns and problems. Concrete examples should be provided. Present one concept at a time, and allow time for processing that information. Utilize repetition and reinforcement by providing written instructions. When using written instructions, make sure they are appropriate for the students' literacy level and possible visual impairments. Keep explanations brief; use analogies and visual aids during explanations. Demonstrate the relevance of the presented information to the students' daily life. Try to identify positive past experiences and relate them to the presented information.

Teaching clients with low literacy levels

Working with this type of client will require the instructor to use innovative and alternative strategies in order to break down this barrier to learning. Examples of such strategies include:
- The teacher should establish trust before beginning the teaching-learning process by getting to know the client and focusing on their strengths.
- Teach one simple step at a time to help reduce client anxiety and confusion.
- Use methods and tools which do not require many pre-existing literacy skills.
- Explain information in concrete, simple terms reflecting the client's language skills.
- Make the information as simple as possible to teach what the client must learn.
- Allow the client an opportunity to restate the information in their own words to exhibit their understanding of the material. Methods the client can use to show comprehension include demonstration, hands-on practice, and role-play.
- Use repetition to help reinforce the material. All major points should be reviewed. It is advantageous for this type of student to have the same material repeated in different ways.

Clients with low socioeconomic status

The nurse educator must be careful to avoid stereotyping individuals, particularly based on their socioeconomic status. However, there is often a correlation between low socioeconomic status and poor cognitive functioning and academic achievement, less availability of social support systems, decreased literacy, and increased susceptibility to disease. It is necessary to assess each individual to ascertain their strengths and weaknesses with regard to learning. The low SES student will generally tend to think in more concrete terms, have a decreased attention span, be more focused on their immediate needs being met, and will tend to view themselves as having an external locus of control. Problem-solving skills and the ability to analyze and interpret large amounts of educational material may be lacking.

Categories of effective teaching

The six basic categories of effective teaching in nursing are:

- Professional competence — The teacher must have excellent skills from personal experience in his/her career, as well as a thorough knowledge of the material. The teacher should read, research, perform clinical practice, and maintain continuing education to continually broaden his/her understanding of the subject matter.
- Personal characteristics — Those characteristics most desirable in an effective educator are: a good speaking voice, confidence, empathy, enthusiasm, genuineness, positive attitude, a sense of humor, flexibility, and patience.
- Relationship with students — An effective educator has a good relationship with his or her students. Educators can enhance this relationship by practicing three therapeutic approaches: empathetic listening, acceptance, and truthful communication.
- Teaching practices — These practices include the mechanics, skills, and methods used in the classroom and the clinical setting. The material should be well-organized and presented in an interesting way.
- Availability to students — The instructor should be available to his/her students when needed.
- Evaluation practices — Expectations should be communicated simply, and feedback should be provided in a timely manner.

Teaching strategies

Activity-based
Activity-based teaching strategies, or methods based around students performing tasks, include cooperative learning, simulations, games and case studies, problem-based learning, and self-learning modules. Cooperative learning involves group projects in which each student is responsible for the learning of all group members. Simulations and games generally involve an exercise in role-playing. Problem-based learning is conducted within a small group of students presented with a real-life problem in which they analyze the case, identify required information, and solve the problem. A self-learning module allows student independence in achieving learning outcomes by utilizing learning materials at their own pace.

<u>Traditional</u>
In comparison, traditional teaching strategies include lecturing, class discussion, questioning, use of audiovisual materials, and the interactive lecture. The class discussion strategy may be formal or informal, often starting when the teacher asks, "Are there any questions?" The questioning strategy is utilized by asking a simple or complex question. Audiovisual materials may involve utilizing overhead projectors, watching a DVD, or writing on the chalkboard. The interactive lecture involves combining several of the above strategies.

Computer technology as a teaching tool

<u>Advantages</u>
Computers support mastery learning well. The student is able to spend as much time as necessary in order to master learning concepts and skills. A student can generally access a computer for a greater length of time than his/her teacher. Computers can assist in maximizing time spent in learning a task. Computers can motivate the student to spend more time mastering the objectives through interesting programming and more varied methods of learning. Instant feedback on the student's progress, an effective learning tool, can be provided. Additionally, computers are objective and nonjudgmental with feedback. Some other advantages of using computer instruction are consistency of instruction, reduction of repetitive teacher tasks, personalized instruction, cost effectiveness, and time efficiency. Using computer instruction, the student is able to maintain control of the learning process by manipulating the speed, order, and type of instruction.

<u>Disadvantages</u>
Some teachers feel uncomfortable utilizing computer instruction. These instructors may not have good computer skills, or they may have difficulty knowing how to utilize computers in their instruction. Busy educators may not feel they have the time to learn new technologies. Another potential disadvantage is the lack of face-to-face interaction between the student, the teacher, and the patient. Nurses must be trained to interpret nonverbal communication in a social setting to obtain an accurate assessment when performing nursing tasks. Another concern is the time required to learn complex technologies that may differ from setting to setting. Different hospitals may utilize different computer systems, requiring the student to spend time learning a new system. The time required may, in turn, subtract from direct patient contact time.

Gagne's hierarchy of learning

Gagne's hierarchy of learning consists of eight different types:
- Signal Learning: The student exhibits a conditioned response to a stimulus, such as becoming nervous when the word "test" is used.
- Stimulus-Response Learning: The student develops a voluntary response to a stimulus as taught by the instructor.

- Chaining: This is a series of conditioned responses which are related, generally in a logical or sequential fashion.
- Verbal Association: This is a type of chaining where the student associates new subject matter with older, previously learned subject matter or terms. In this way, the new material or terminology is learned more easily.
- Discrimination Learning: The student discriminates between large amounts of new information by finding something unique about each, so that retention can be increased.
- Concept Learning: The student learns how to classify information into groups delineated by a shared concept.
- Rule Learning: Rules are generally expressed by "If...then" statements, which express relationships between concepts.
- Problem Solving: This is the most complex form of learning. It is a process of understanding both the problem and the goal being sought. The rules the student has learned must be recalled and applied in order to solve the problem.

Teaching psychomotor skills

The elements of effective skill demonstrations which would be utilized when teaching psychomotor skills to the nursing student or the patient are as follows:
- Prepare and assemble all needed equipment before the demonstration.
- Check that all equipment works.
- Practice the procedure, and determine the time the demonstration will take.
- Prepare the environment to be as realistic as possible.Each step as the procedure is performed.
- Give the rationale for each action when it is appropriate.
- In order to show fine points which may not be discernible by the students or patients, refer to written materials such as handouts and/or textbooks.
- Always practice the principles of good nursing care while performing the demonstration.
- Either perform the skill a second time, or have a student perform without inserting explanations, in order to show the proper flow of the skill.

Reflective thinking practices

One of the best ways to incorporate reflective thinking practices in the learning environment is to encourage the student, patient, or colleague to record their learning experiences in a journal; whether it is a handwritten journal or an electronic journal on the computer. This allows the student or instructor to think more deeply on the subject matter, and their assumptions will be recorded and acknowledged. Journal writing allows the student to interpret and make sense of the information. This allows the information to be built into the previous knowledge base, and creates a fresh interpretation of the information. Journal writing is also a way to show what the student knows and comprehends. Questions may arise which might not have occurred to the student during the actual experience. This allows the instructor to assess what the student knows, as well as the assumptions about what they have learned. Reflective practice groups utilizing discussion among peers can be incorporated among teaching colleagues to assist them in reflecting on their own professional practice as well.

Among educational colleagues
Educator learning is supported by participation in reflective practice groups. The instructor, with colleagues, may explore assumptions which guide their thinking and thus, their behaviors. This may promote an understanding of how their assumptions affect their problem solving. By examining his/her own assumptions, the instructor can bring lasting change and develop new practices. Events can be paused and reviewed by the group. Other ways of thinking and reacting can be explored by the group. Reflective thinking practices can provide a safe environment for exploring the educators' own assumptions and beliefs. By participating in this practice on a regular basis, educators can facilitate their professional development and learning.

Critical thinking

As defined by the National League of Nurses, critical thinking in the nursing practice is "a discipline specific, reflective reasoning process that guides a nurse in generating, implementing, and evaluating approaches for dealing with client care and professional concerns."

Some tools used to assess critical thinking skills are as follows:
- Several standardized tests are used to evaluate critical thinking skills. These tests include: California Critical Thinking Skills Test (CCTST), California Critical Thinking Dispositions Inventory (CCTDI), Watson-Glaser Critical Thinking Appraisal (WGCTA), Learning Environment Preference Test (LEP), and the Critical Thinking in Clinical Nursing Practice/RN Test.
- Some other tools and methodologies used include: having the student develop a concept map on a particular topic; examining their learning portfolio; evaluating their laboratory performance; and observing the behaviors of the student, such as:
  o Ability to accept those with different viewpoints.
  o Realization that every student has their own opinions and inclinations.
  o Ability to delay or amend their problem-solving when presented with either the absence of enough information or new information.

Strategies to strengthen skills
The following strategies can provide students with methods and opportunities to develop and strengthen critical thinking skills:
- Concept Mapping: Causes the students to evaluate on paper what they know about a given situation, and examine how all the pieces of the puzzle need to fit in order to solve the problem.

- Problem-Based Learning: Used by a group of students working as a team. The team is presented with a clinical-type problem which needs to be addressed and solved utilizing various resources available to them.
- Text Interaction: Applied when the student reads the textbook assignment prior to class and thinks critically about the information presented.
- Effective Questioning: Allows the teacher to ask questions which require a thoughtful answer, allowing the students to evaluate and consider their own, as well as differing, viewpoints.
- Discussion: Involves thoughtful dialogue between a teacher and his/her students. The teacher may model critical thinking by "thinking out loud" to demonstrate how to arrive at a conclusion.

Some other strategies include, but are not limited to: case studies, focused reflection, service learning, self-assessment, and collaborative learning.

Limitations

By entertaining incorrect assumptions about beginning nursing students, educators can limit their ability to think critically. Some incorrect assumptions are: the students are unable or do not know how to problem solve; the faculty knows best; there is a single most certain way to think about or find solutions; and mistakes are negative and should always be avoided. By relying on the lecture as the major method of educating; the nursing student becomes passive in the process. Class material that is presented in a manner that is too structured or overly simplified may cause students to incorrectly interpret the material as uncomplicated and easily manageable. The assignments given students often do not appeal to their critical thinking skills. Tests and assessments are often too concrete, with no need for the student to practice complex thinking.

Positive learning environment

A positive learning environment is an atmosphere of respect, support, and a feeling of safety. The instructor should provide a proper balance of challenge and support in this environment. Silence can be utilized by the instructor to encourage reflection by the student. Instructors should provide support by guiding their students, providing structure, giving them good examples, and providing opportunities to have real-life experiences. The student should feel unafraid to take risks, because they will often learn the most by making some mistakes. The instructor can strive to minimize the pain of possibly making a mistake in this type of setting. The educator's role should be supporting and encouraging; instructors should assist the students in organizing their knowledge, skills, and attitudes. In this way, the students may reach their greatest potential.

The educator has the ability to set the tone for the class during the very first meeting. The initial impressions made by the educator will set the tone and can be used to establish a positive learning environment. During the initial meeting, instructors should introduce themselves and identify how they prefer the students to address them. They should also share some personal or professional information about themselves. If appropriate, finding a way to inject humor will create a pleasant atmosphere. Welcome the class and read names to obtain correct pronunciations. Expectations should be communicated. The course syllabus should be reviewed. Allow time to take questions. Cover general classroom rules. Discuss how the information they are about to learn will help them, and how they will be able to apply it practically to their lives. Try to communicate enthusiasm for the material the students are about to learn. After the initial class, it is important to gain and control the attention of the students. The educator should always convey being in control of the classroom.

<u>Relationship with clinical agency personnel</u>
A collegial working relationship should be established with clinical agency personnel in order to promote a positive learning environment. Extensive planning on the part of the instructor prior to the clinical experience must be accomplished. The instructor is instrumental in gathering information necessary to develop a written contract between the educational institution and the clinical agency. Contract details may include: the availability of conference space and the clinical unit for specified days, the ratio of students to faculty, and evidence of required malpractice and liability insurance for the faculty and students. The educator should arrange a meeting with the clinical agency staff who will be involved with the learning process.
Learning objectives can be discussed and agreed upon. Student assignments of patients should be done prior to the laboratory experience with the input of clinical staff members.

Evidence-based practice

Evidence-based practice in nursing means integrating research with clinical expertise and patient values, while making the best decisions about patient care. To utilize evidence-based practice, the instructor must direct the student to follow five basic steps. First, the student should develop a well-formulated question. Second, articles and other research material that address the question should be identified. Next, the evidence should be critically appraised to determine its validity. The evidence should then be applied to the issue at hand. Finally, the application of this evidence should be evaluated, and areas of improvement should be identified.

Information-processing model of memory

The information-processing model of memory is a multi-stage construct, where the first stage of the information processing model of memory is the student's ability to pay attention to their surroundings and outside input. Sensory information is processed in the next stage of the model. During the third stage, the information is built into short-term memory. This brief incorporation of information will result in either discarding or storing the learned material in long-term memory. In the final stage, the student will perform tasks based on processed and stored information.

Each stage of information processing can be affected by various factors. If in the initial stage, the student is unable to pay attention to outside stimuli due to fatigue, distraction, or the effects of medication, etc., information processing will not begin at all. During the second stage, the student could have sensory deficits, or their preferred mode of processing information may differ from how the material is presented. The third stage of processing can be adversely affected by the difficulty in retrieving that stored information.

Effective teaching tools

Computer-assisted instruction, or CAI, is a method of self-paced study utilizing computer technology, which is individualized to present a specific instructional activity. This method is useful in reinforcing cognitive learning. The ability of this instructional method to teach effectively depends on the student's motivation to adequately utilize this type of technology. The instructional software and hardware must be technologically adequate as well.

Audio learning resources include such tools as audiotapes and recorders. The main purpose of such tools is to provide instruction by utilizing the students' sense of hearing as a mechanism for learning.

Audiovisual materials include any instructional media which can influence learning and appeal to the students' senses of hearing and/or sight. Materials may include any of the following: telecommunications, computer formats, video, audio, or projected visual presentations, such as from an overhead projector.

Gardner's intelligence types

Gardner's eight types of intelligence and effective teaching strategies that apply to each type are:
- Linguistic intelligence: Students exhibit highly developed auditory skills. Oral quizzes, lectures, giving directions out loud, and utilizing study and discussion groups work well for this student.
- Logical mathematical intelligence: Students exhibit logical thinking with a high degree of abstraction. Teaching methods for this type include utilizing reasoning activities and grouping concepts into categories.
- Spatial intelligence: Students learn best by illustrations and images. Charts and diagrams work well for this student.
- Musical intelligence: Students often process information best with music playing in the background.
- Bodily kinesthetic intelligence: Students must process knowledge by moving around, role play and utilizing manipulating objects.

- Interpersonal intelligence: Students understand people and are sensitive to others' emotions. Group learning and group problem-solving promote their learning.
- Intrapersonal intelligence: Students prefer their own inner world of feelings and ideas. Independent, self-directed study work best for these individuals.
- Naturalistic intelligence: Students are able to make patterns and connections to the elements of nature. They learn best by engaging with nature. Pet therapy and nature walks are good methods to utilize.

Learning style

Instruments to determine style
Instruments used to assess left-brain/right-brain and whole-brain thinking includes the BPI, or brain preference indicator, and the HBDI, or Herrmann brain dominance instrument. The GEFT, or Group Embedded Figures Test, is used to measure field independence/dependence. This instrument assesses the student's ability to discover basic geometric shapes within a more complex illustration. The Dunn and Dunn learning style inventory identifies how a student prefers to perform, function, and study. The adult version is called the PEPS, or Productivity Environmental Preference Survey. This tool indicates learning preference. The MBTI, or Myers-Briggs Type Indicator, helps students understand how they interact with others with regard to their personality type. This can assist the educator in understanding students' preferences in learning by how they perceive and judge information. The Learning Style Inventory, or LSI, requires the test-taker to answer a 12-item questionnaire, which should help to categorize their learning style as a doer, feeler, thinker, or watcher.

Style principles described by Friedman and Alley
The six learning styles, as described by Friedman and Alley, are as follows:
- Both the style by which the educator prefers to teach and the style by which the student prefers to learn can be identified.
- Educators need to guard against relying on teaching methods and tools that match their own preferred learning styles.
- Educators are most helpful when they assist students in identifying and learning through their own style preferences.
- Students should have the opportunity to learn through their preferred style.
- Students should be encouraged to diversify their style preferences.
- Educators can develop specific learning activities that reinforce each modality or style.

Purnell's cultural domains

The twelve cultural domains identified by the Purnell model are: communication; family roles and organization; workforce issues; biocultural ecology, such as genetics and heredity; high-risk behaviors, such as smoking and alcoholism;

nutrition; pregnancy; death rituals; spirituality; health care practices; health care practitioners, such as gender issues and perception of providers; and cultural heritage, such as occupation, economics, and education.

Nurse educators must familiarize themselves with cultural characteristics of clients from different backgrounds. They should create a trusting environment in which the patient can discuss their unique needs and freely express themselves. Differences in cultures and their belief systems must be understood. The educator should ask questions regarding these belief systems, such as "What do you think caused your problem?" and "What do you fear most about your illness?" Utilizing a translator may prove beneficial. Some other examples of effective teaching strategies are: provide enough space for teaching in order to involve family members; speak slowly and clearly; avoid using technical terms and English slang; and provide teaching materials in the client's native language.

Acting as role model

One of the ways a nurse educator may be an effective role model is by keeping abreast of the most up-to-date information. This can be achieved by actively maintaining continuing education in the field of nursing, particularly in their area of expertise. This can be accomplished by subscribing to professional journals and attending seminars. Instructors should engage in scholarly activities, such as performing research and writing professional papers. Additionally, educators should obtain advanced credentials. There should always be agreement between what the teacher says and does. Finally, the instructor should exhibit positive enthusiasm regarding the subject matter. In this way, the student will model an enthusiasm for learning and in the practice of the newly acquired skill.

Models of clinical teaching

Advantages and disadvantages
The traditional clinical teaching model in nursing education has been the assignment of a group of 8-12 nursing students to an instructor who accompanies them to a clinical agency site. These students are then assigned to patients in order to provide hands-on care in the clinical setting. The advantage of this model is that it provides experience with real-life patient care in a real clinical environment (hospital setting). Some disadvantages of this model include the inability of the instructor to provide equal attention to each student due to the unpredictable nature of the hospital setting. Since the instructor is a guest at the institution and not an actual staff member, she/he may not be familiar with all of their culture and policies. This may cause a lack of trust by the actual staff members of the institution, possibly leading to a real feeling of disconnect between the instructor and the staff.

Other models

Having the nursing students remain in a skills laboratory until they have mastered a particular skill, or group of skills, is a different model that has been used with success. Once these skills have been mastered, the students are sent out to practice only their learned psychomotor skill in the clinical setting. Another model proposes that more information is provided in the classroom before the students go to the clinical laboratory or the clinical agency. This course incorporates small groups of students who utilize case studies and questioning. This allows practice involving "real-life situations" in the safety of the classroom setting. The instructor would be able to guide students in developing and practicing such skills as decision-making, prioritizing, time management, delegation, and appropriate communication among other professionals. Preceptorship is another model utilized in both undergraduate and graduate nursing student programs. In this model, a preceptor is assigned to supervise and guide individual students. This preceptor is a practicing nurse employed by the clinical agency.

Electronic communication with health care consumers

Educators can communicate electronically through the use of e-mail, discussion or Usenet newsgroups, or real-time chat. This provides easy access to communication between the consumer and the professional. It also provides an excellent way to follow up in regard to questions which may occur after leaving the clinical setting. It allows follow up to assess a proper understanding of discharge instructions and compliance. The consumer has time to compose their thoughts and questions outside of the clinic atmosphere, where they may often feel rushed or intimidated. However, it is not practical when there are urgent medical needs, as it may come across as unfeeling to the patient. The nurse will not have the ability to use non-verbal aspects of communication, such as facial expressions or tone of voice. It provides a written record of instructions and advice given, so the response must be carefully reviewed for accuracy and thoughtfulness. Protection of the patient's medical privacy can be at risk when utilizing this type of communication.

Principles of good practice

The seven principles of good practice in undergraduate education, as proposed by Chickering and Gamson are as follows:
- Encourage student-faculty contact. This should include student-faculty contact outside of class time. Ideally, instructors should be rewarded by their employing institutions for extra time spent with students.
- Encourage cooperation among students. This should include time spent learning collaboratively, rather than competitively.
- Encourage active learning. Instructors should promote active rather than passive learning in their students.
- Give prompt feedback. This enhances and facilitates learning.

- Emphasize time on task. Students should be coached to take studying seriously. Time management skills should be promoted in regards to how much time to spend on various learning tasks.
- Communicate high expectations. Students should be motivated and encouraged to meet their instructor's high expectations.
- Respect diverse talents and ways of learning. Instructors should be aware of, and take into consideration, students' different learning styles.

Learning theories

The five main learning theories are:
- Behaviorist Learning: This model may also be referred to as the S-R model of learning. It is learning accomplished through the product of stimulus conditions (S) and the responses (R) resulting from that stimulus. The learning focus is on what is directly observable.
- Cognitive Learning: Students change due to the way they perceive, process, interpret, and organize the new information and how they incorporate it into what they already know. This will lead to new insights and comprehension.
- Psychodynamic Learning: Conscious and unconscious forces in the student, caused by earlier experiences and conflicts, will help guide and modify behavior.
- Social Learning: A central concept to this theory is role modeling. The student is believed to observe and watch the behavior of others and the results that occur from that behavior. This is a social process that combines behaviorist, cognitive, and psychodynamic learning.
- Humanistic Learning: This learning is produced through a combination of curiosity, positive self-concept, and the student's needs. The student is given a freedom of choice. Their uniqueness is honored and encouraged.

Instruction/learning methods

Group discussion
One of the major advantages of this method is it stimulates students to seriously think about specific issues and difficult situations. A free exchange of ideas is encouraged. Life experiences can be shared among the student. Learning thus becomes more active, and peer support and a sense of group belonging is promoted. An instructive group setting allows the educator to reach many students at the same time. This can prove to be economically beneficial.

Some problems with this method can include the possibility of certain clients to take control of the discussion and not allow for shy or introverted members to participate. The possibility of getting off topic is real. This method can prove to be more time-consuming than other methods of learning. The teacher must always be present to act as the group facilitator.

Lecture

One of the major advantages of this method is that it provides an efficient, economical way to transmit a lot of information to a large group of people within a short time frame. This method can highlight patterns and main ideas in the material. It can provide the information needed to facilitate a later discussion group. It can help to summarize research findings in a more understandable manner.

Some limitations include the role of the student as passive when utilizing this method. It often is unable to appeal to all students, due to their different backgrounds and learning styles. Thus, the ability to reach all students equally is inhibited.

Demonstration and return demonstration

This method engages the student by stimulating the auditory, visual, and tactile senses. The student is taught within the psychomotor domain. Retention of the skill is enhanced through repetition and reinforcement. This increases the confidence and competence of the student. Since the student is allowed to utilize the equipment and perform the procedure prior to the actual experience, this will reduce their anxiety level when actual performance is required.

However, this is a time-intensive method. In order for this method to be effective, the size of the learning group must be kept small. Extra space and expensive equipment to perform these demonstrations may be required.

Self-instruction

This method promotes active, as opposed to passive, learning. It allows students to set their own pace. The student has time to frequently review the information and reflect upon it, and is provided with frequent feedback, which is built into the method.

Some possible disadvantages of this method entail the fact that it is not universally beneficial for every student. Some students will have difficulty with the traditional method of self-instruction, due to hearing or visual impairments. It is not the ideal approach for the patient with a low literacy level. The student must be self-motivated and not be a procrastinator. This method can prove boring for some students over time.

One-to-one instruction

The one-to-one instruction method works well for students with learning disabilities, low education levels, and/or low literacy levels. This method is useful when initially assessing the student's abilities, and for the evaluation of learning on an ongoing basis. The pace of learning can be individualized to meet the student's demands.

There are some limitations to this method. It lacks the opportunity for the student to be able to identify and share information, emotions, and thoughts with others in similar situations. It can prove more stressful to the student, due to the fact they are receiving the teacher's full attention. This method is labor-intensive, and thus proves to be inefficient from an economic standpoint.

Role-playing and role-modeling
For role-playing to be effective, the group must feel comfortable enough to act out a particular situation in a realistic manner. This method allows individuals to explore their own feelings and attitudes about the situation. It allows the students to see and understand a complex situation from another perspective. Role-modeling allows instructors to demonstrate behaviors they would like modeled by their students. By providing a positive role model, the desired behaviors can be reproduced in the student.
In order for role-playing to be an effective method, it must be performed in a small group situation. If the role is played too dramatically, it will lose its believability and the activity will prove to be ineffective. Some students will feel too uncomfortable to accurately play their roles. Similarly, some limitations of role-modeling include the fact that negative role models do exist. This creates the potential to cause unacceptable behaviors in the student. There must be a positive relationship between the student and role model.

Audiovisual tools

In order for the AV materials to be effective, the instructor should be familiar with the content before it is utilized. The AV tools should enhance and reinforce the instruction provided by the educator. The media should coincide with and help to accomplish the learning objectives, and should fall within the given budget. The information provided by the AV material should be current and accurate, as well as unbiased. The material should be appropriate given the age, physical abilities, and educational level of the student. The five major categories include: telecommunications, computer formats, video, audio, and projected audiovisual tools.

Faculty development

Adult learning principles
The six adult learning principles as they relate to faculty development, as proposed by Lawler and King (2000), are as follows:
- Create a climate of respect: The faculty educator should understand that each faculty member has their own viewpoint and unique experiences to share and offer to the learning group.
- Encourage active participation: By encouraging active participation in the educational process, the faculty member is valued as having something to offer the entire learning group.

- Build on experience: Adult students have a variety of past experiences. The acceptance of new information relies on incorporating it with prior experiences.
- Employ collaborative inquiry: To encourage collaborative inquiry, faculty members' input should be sought with regard to planning the educational experience.
- Learn for action: Faculty members should be encouraged to incorporate and put the new material learned into action. The educator should create a supportive environment among faculty members for experimentation with and practice of the newly learned information.
- Empower participants: When the faculty members incorporate the new information within their prior experiences; change will occur. They will be empowered by this new change and understanding.

Main tasks during the planning stage

The faculty program developer should complete the following tasks during the planning stage:
- Selecting a topic: A needs assessment should be accomplished and program objectives should be established. Content and topic areas should be identified.
- Identifying a presenter: Research should be accomplished with regard to experts available in the identified field of study. The experts should be considered credible by the faculty members.
- Preparing for delivery: Materials should be prepared and the curriculum should be developed to meet the established objectives.
- Preparing for support and transfer of learning: Program developers should determine what resources and support are available to promote a transfer learning among faculty before, during, and after the learning activity.
- Scheduling the event: The program timing and availability must be practical to meet the faculty members' needs.
- Beginning the evaluation: The developer must focus on what will be evaluated during and after the program's completion.

Domains of learning

The *cognitive domain* is also known as the thinking domain. Learning in this domain involves knowledge and comprehension. This domain is what teaching has traditionally been most focused upon. The instructor acts as the "giver of information" in this type of learning. The student must be able to apply, analyze, synthesize, and evaluate this knowledge.

The *affective domain* is also known as the feeling domain. This type of learning involves internalizing the new information. Teaching methods in this domain include role modeling, simulation, group discussion, and role playing. Learning in this domain involves accepting, responding to, valuing, organizing, and characterizing the new information.

The *psychomotor domain* is also known as the skills domain. This type of learning involves developing fine and gross motor skills. Some teaching methods include demonstration and return demonstration, as well as mental imaging. Steps to learning in this domain include observing, imitating, practicing, and adapting.

Illiteracy

Common myths
Three common myths exist about people who are illiterate. They are often assumed to have a low IQ, be incapable of learning or be slow students. In actuality, they usually have an average or above average IQ. It is also assumed they are easily identified by their appearance. However, articulate, well-dressed people can have no outward signs of illiteracy and still be illiterate. Furthermore, it is often assumed that the number of school years completed will correlate with literacy.

Behavioral clues
The most important thing to remember in recognizing illiteracy is there is no stereotype. Nurses should never assume that their clients are literate. Some possible behaviors which may be demonstrated by a person with low literacy are as follows. The person may react to a complex learning situation by withdrawing or avoidance. They may be noncompliant. They may ask for the information to be read to them, due to various complaints and excuses. They may appear confused, nervous, frustrated, or restless when attempting to read, or may hold the material upside down.

Permanent learning

Learning will have a tendency to become permanent if the educator is able to organize the experience, make it meaningful and pleasurable, recognize the role of emotions in learning, and follow an appropriate pace, which allows the student to process the material. The student must have the ability to practice the learned knowledge or skills. Reinforcement of the knowledge or skill will cause it to become more permanently learned. Learning must be measured soon after the experience, as well as at later times, to determine its permanence. The educator can then take this feedback and reorganize or revitalize the learning experience to cause more reinforcement and permanent retention.

Teaching styles

Teaching style is a blend of the educator's personality, character, and intellect. It goes beyond having certain behaviors or skills. Some various unique teaching styles may include the following aspects: humor, a pleasant tone or speaking voice, animated gestures, talented timing in delivery, the ability to understand the needs of the classroom (such as when to spend more time explaining a particular topic), and the incorporation of story-telling as a teaching tool. There are generally two main types of teaching styles: the student centered approach and the teacher centered approach. The teacher centered style views the students as passive students. These teachers may focus more on teaching the students than assessing their learning and comprehension. The student centered approach incorporates a collaborative relationship between the educator and the student. This style generally seeks to cause students to utilize critical thinking skills.

Important terms

Ethnic group: A population of people also referred to as a subculture, which has different experiences from those of the dominant culture.

Ethnocentrism: A concept in which the belief is held that one's own culture is superior and all other cultures are less sophisticated.

Assimilation: The willingness of a person emigrating to a new culture to gradually adopt and incorporate the characteristics of the prevailing culture.

Acculturation: scribes an individual's adaptation to the customs, values, beliefs, and behaviors of a new country or culture.

Culture: A complex concept that is an integral part of each person's life and includes knowledge, beliefs, values, morals, customs, traditions, and habits acquired by the members of a society.

Blog: This is becoming a very popular mechanism for information sharing online about a particular topic by individuals. Individuals write responses and ideas on a particular topic which can be viewed by others. Blogs are also known as Web logs or Web diaries.

E-learning: This is an abbreviation for electronic learning. It utilizes computer technology to provide educational materials, and provides customized learning anytime or anywhere. E-learning can be very beneficial in providing training to the workforce.

Distance learning: This technology utilizes video or computer technology through the use of telecommunications to provide live, online, or taped information between the student and instructor, who are separated by location or time.

Digital divide: This is a term used to describe the difference between those individuals who have access to information technology resources and those who do not.

World Wide Web: This is a technology-based learning resource which is virtual space specifically for the display of information. It represents a computer network of information servers throughout the world connected through the Internet.

Internet: This global computer network was established to allow the exchange of information from one computer to another. Some examples of communication facilitated through the Internet include e-mail, real-time chat, and electronic discussion groups.

Information Age: This term represents the present period of time. This period has involved major advances in information and computer technology. This has transformed our society economically, socially, and culturally.

Consumer informatics: This particular discipline analyzes the consumers' information needs. A computer informatics researcher studies and implements ways to make information accessible, and models and integrates this information.

Determinants of learning: This refers to what factors influence how well an individual learns. The three determinants of learning that must be assessed by the educator are the students' needs, readiness to learn, and their preferred learning style. Some initial steps to take in order to assess a student's needs are as follows: determine who composes your audience, choose the best setting, collect data about and from the student, involve members of the health care team, and prioritize needs.

Readiness to learn: This refers to the time that the student is receptive, willing, and able to participate in the educational process. When a student asks a question, this often signifies a readiness to learn.

Learning style: This is the way the students learn, taking into account the cognitive, affective, and physiological factors that affect how students perceive, interact with, and respond to the learning environment.

Facilitate Learner Development

Assessing student needs

In order to develop an appropriate educational program or experience, the needs of the student must be explored and identified. In this way, the student's needs are addressed appropriately. Optimal learning will occur with the least amount of anxiety for the student. A proper assessment can reduce unnecessary repetition, utilize time more efficiently, and develop a positive rapport between teacher and student. When performing a needs assessment, the educator must assess the main determinants of learning. These include the learning needs, the readiness to learn, and the student's learning style. The assessment phase is most often overlooked because of lack of time. For this reason, the nurse educator must continually be aware of the three determinants in the assessment of the student. In this way, necessary learning can be conducted in a timely, organized, efficient manner.

Methods

Nurse educators must collect objective and subjective information about their students in order to assess their learning needs. In order to obtain the most extensive information, several methods should be utilized concurrently. Information can be gathered through informal conversations. Educators can ask open-ended questions and use active listening skills to gather valuable information. A structured interview may be performed by the educator. The client is interviewed in person or by telephone to assess their needs. By utilizing a focus group, the instructor can gather information by facilitating discussion among a group of 4-12 students. Self-administered questionnaires can be made available to the potential students. The educator should encourage the responders to be honest, and additional concerns should be solicited. Tests and pretests are valuable assessment methods. Observations and review of patient charts are also excellent assessment methods. The student's health behaviors or performance of a psychomotor skill can be observed. Reviewing the chart for information shared by other professionals may also prove helpful.

Hearing-impaired students

The hearing-impaired student will need to rely on other senses to obtain information. Most commonly, such students will rely upon their visual sense. Communication should be visible to this type of student. Depending on when deafness occurred and its duration, the learning needs will vary. The educator will need to identify this student's preferred method of communication. Methods may include some or all of the following: sign language, written materials, lip reading, sound augmentation, telecommunications, and verbalization by the client. For most deaf clients who know American Sign Language, this will be the method of choice.

The nurse educator will need to obtain a professional interpreter or the assistance of a family member to assist with this form of communication. If the student is attempting to lip-read, sufficient lighting should be provided and other forms of communication should supplement this method, as less than half of the English language is able to be lip-read. Written materials are considered to be the most reliable form of communication, but the student must be literate.

Visually-impaired students

The nurse educator will want to investigate the most appropriate learning methods for their visually-impaired clients. A client who has had a long-standing history of visual impairment will be able to share what has worked well in the past. This type of client will generally have a heightened acuity of the other senses. The most common senses utilized are the auditory and tactile senses. The instructor should be aware of the need to verbally explain things that are normally taken for granted, such as one's presence, as well as colors, shapes, and nonverbal language cues. Audio learning devices, such as cassettes and compact discs, are great tools. Computers that have synthetic speech or Braille are excellent. Utilizing written materials in Braille is helpful. For those that have diminished vision, enlarging print and good lighting will be helpful. Providing contrast or colors will also be helpful in distinguishing objects visually.

Support and assistance for diverse students

One way to support and assist the diverse student is to have an increase in minority representation in nursing. Nurses should be educated to value and respect multicultural and multiracial viewpoints. They should strive to understand the cultural characteristics and traits of the students. Nurses should foster an environment which promotes a feeling of acceptance in the diverse patient. The students should feel comfortable expressing their feelings, ideas, and sharing their unique needs. The nursing curriculum should strive to incorporate social values that acknowledge these different perspectives and lifestyles. In this way, the nurses who are educated to teach such students will respect their differences and handle them in a professional and appropriate manner.

Purnell's cultural domains

The 12 cultural domains should be assessed when instructors are planning education for students in a variety of settings. These domains are as follows:
- Communication should be examined. This includes the student's dominant language, as well as nonverbal cues.
- Family roles and its organization should be considered. This might include the student's social status or gender roles.
- Workforce issues are assessed.
- Biocultural ecology or heredity should be assessed.

- The student's high-risk behaviors, such as smoking or physical activity, should be evaluated.
- Nutrition is assessed. This includes common foods eaten, as well as rituals or limitations practiced.
- Pregnancy beliefs and views should be examined.
- Death rituals need to be respected. Views of death and bereavement practices should be acknowledged.
- Spirituality must be honored and understood.
- Health care practices need to be considered. Pain control and the view of their health responsibility should be assessed.
- Perceptions of health care practitioners should be understood.
- The student's heritage should be studied and valued.

Learning needs of nursing staff

The nurse educator should obtain learning needs information from various sources in the clinical setting. Some sources include: performance evaluations, incident reports, nursing staff input, interviews with nurse managers, quality improvement reports, and nursing audits. There may be additional needs of the staff that can arise out of their personal demands and situations at home. This may, for example, affect their availability to attend continuing education programs after work hours. Distance education programs and self-directed study programs can be most beneficial for these staff members. Characteristics of staff members must be taken into consideration in the development of learning programs. Some characteristics include prior education, previous work experience, and their present knowledge and skills with respect to what is needed to perform at their optimal level.

Teaching styles and affect on behaviors

A teaching style that incorporates positive feedback and provides it frequently will cause the praised behavior to be repeated by the student. A teaching style which does not provide feedback to the student may promote poor habits. The student may practice the skill they wish to accomplish regularly, but without external feedback and correction or redirection from their instructor, they may practice it incorrectly and develop poor or incorrect habits. A teaching style that threatens punishment for mistakes may actually inhibit further learning by causing nervousness and avoidance in the student.

A teaching style that provides immediate feedback to the student is much more effective than a style that provides delayed feedback. When the student has immediate knowledge of their success, they are able to continue to learn more material. A teaching style that motivates students can encourage them to rise above mediocrity. By invoking the students' curiosity and desire to improve their quality of life, the teacher can motivate increased learning.

If a person believes that he or she can accomplish a task, he or she is more likely to work and persevere to learn the task. The nurse educator can be instrumental in providing opportunities for the client or student to learn by doing. The student will develop performance accomplishments by having successful experiences of learning by doing. The instructor can also increase a student's belief in his or her own abilities to accomplish a task by providing opportunities for watching someone else perform the behavior successfully. This is termed vicarious experience or learning through observation. The instructor can often serve as this "someone" or model. The educator can also facilitate learning or behavior change by providing encouragement to the student or client who is attempting to master a behavior or task. This is termed verbal persuasion.

Social cognitive theory
This theory states that a behavior is the result of an interaction among self, environment, and the behavior. The theory proposes that a change in one of these factors affects all of them; this theory is also known as reciprocal determinism. Role modeling is an essential concept of this theory, and can be incorporated to facilitate learning. Nurse educators, managers, and preceptors all have the opportunity to role model and thus utilize this theory in effecting behavior change and ultimately learning in the nursing student. Learning becomes a social process when incorporating this theory. Role modeling can also be provided by a family member, another patient, or the instructor, so the student can model the sought-after new behavior. By observing others perform the behavior successfully; the student will adopt a positive attitude and belief in their ability to accomplish the new behavior.

Psychomotor skills

Gentile model of learning
In Gentile's model, there are two main stages: Getting the Idea of the Movement, and Fixation/Diversification. In the first stage, the student must have the ultimate goal in mind and be able to discern between various stimuli which will be experienced during the performance of the skill. The student will have to determine which stimuli are relevant and which are not in accomplishing their psychomotor skill goal. Once the student is able to discern between these various stimuli, he or she must develop a motor plan. This is a visualization of the movements that will be required to accomplish their goal. In the second stage, the student must practice and refine this skill until it is consistent. It is also important to practice the newly learned skill in different or changing environments.

Whole versus part learning
There is debate among educators on what is the best way to teach psychomotor skills. Educators debate whether breaking the skill down into parts or demonstrating the entire skill is the best method. It is generally believed that a more complex skill that involves many steps should be broken down into parts to promote better mastery of the skill. A more simple skill or one whose parts are

interrelated should be taught as a whole. Experienced instructors have an idea of the types of skills that are more difficult for the student to master. The educator can analyze various psychomotor skills to determine their complexity. Time should be spent organizing these more complex skills into appropriate parts. Examples of complex skills that should be divided into parts might include tracheostomy care or starting an intravenous line. Examples of more simple tasks, or those that are interrelated might include a dressing change or vital sign assessment. These tasks should be taught as a whole psychomotor skill.

Independent learning versus teacher instruction

Independent learning of psychomotor skills in a self-directed laboratory environment usually involves the student reviewing various literatures related to the skill and observing recorded demonstrations, as well as other media-portrayed information related to the skill. The students proceed at their own pace. Laboratory instructors are available to assist the students and monitor their testing procedures. Once the skill is accomplished, the students may be given a case scenario in which to perform and adapt their newly learned skill. It has been demonstrated that this type of learning is quite successful. It has actually been demonstrated that students learning by this method often will score higher on cognitive post-tests, as opposed to the group taught the skill only by the instructor. Teacher instruction is much more time-intensive and costly than the independent learning method. There is also a higher chance of error in demonstrations by instructors than a media-portrayed presentation. However, research has revealed that students prefer teacher instruction of psychomotor skills over independent instruction.

The following are terms associated with psychomotor skill learning:
- Regulatory stimuli: External conditions that influence or regulate skill performance and to which the student must pay attention.
- Nonregulatory stimuli: External conditions that do not influence skill performance.
- Closed skill: A skill performed under stable environmental conditions and stimuli.
- Open skill: A skill performed under changing environmental conditions and stimuli.
- Motor plan: A general mental preconception of what movements will be required to perform a skill.
- Fixation: Practicing the skill in the same way each time to fix a reproducible pattern in memory.
- Diversification: Practicing the skill in a variety of ways so that it can be reproduced in a modified way to meet changing environments at any time.
- Arousal: A state of being stirred to action. If arousal is too high, excitability results; if arousal is too low, passivity results.
- Intrinsic feedback: Awareness of performance that arises from within the individual.

- Extrinsic feedback: Awareness of performance that is supplied by an external source.
- Massed practice: Continuously repeated practice sessions with very short or no rest periods between trials.
- Distributed practice: Practice session interspersed with rest periods that are equal to or greater than the practice time.

Bloom's taxonomy

The first level of Bloom's taxonomy is knowledge, which is the ability of the student to memorize, define, or identify various facts, rules, principles and terms. The second level is comprehension, which is the student's ability to demonstrate a comprehension or understanding of the material. The next level is application, which involves the student's ability to utilize the ideas or principles learned in real situations. The fourth level is analysis, in which the student demonstrates the ability to recognize and structure the information. The next level is synthesis, in which the student must take all other levels mastered and put the information together in a unified, demonstrated understanding of the material. The final level is evaluation. The student will be able to judge an action by measuring it against the standards and criteria they have adopted.

Retention of cognitive learning

Most research confirms that learning is best retained when accomplished through several sessions. Learning material through several sessions spaced over time is known as distributed practice. Allowing for set periods of time between sessions will result in more permanent retention of material. For this reason, to successfully perform discharge teaching to the patient, the nurse must not begin on the day of discharge. Discharge teaching should be instituted as soon as feasible during the patient's hospital stay. The same holds true for the student. Teaching material over several sessions and reviewing after some time has passed will produce a higher retention of the learned material.

Affective behavior

Levels
The first level of affective behavior is receiving, wherein the student must demonstrate an awareness of a learned fact. The student must be willing to focus on what is presented. The next level is responding, in which the student is able to respond to an experience. In this level, the student must voluntarily accept the information presented. The third level is known as valuing. The student is now able to accept the worth of the learned theory or idea. Organization is the fourth level, in which the student is able to organize, classify, and prioritize the learned values. The fifth and final level is characterization, in which the student is able to integrate the learned values into a total philosophy or world view.

<u>Affective teaching strategies</u>
Commonly utilized affective teaching strategies practiced by instructors include role playing, role modeling, simulation gaming, and group discussion sessions. These methods assist students in understanding and exploring their attitudes and emotions in relationship to the material presented. These methods assist the student in moving through the five levels of affective behavior. Affective learning in the practicing nurse is important, as she or he is often faced with ethical dilemmas or conflicting values. The educator should provide a relationship of trust and acceptance towards the student. It is important for instructors to dedicate time to teaching in the affective domain, with regard to their nursing students and patients. Some other excellent affective teaching strategies include questioning and the study of various real-life cases.

Faculty development

<u>Adult learning model</u>
The first stage in this model is the pre-planning stage. Organizational goals, climate, and needs are assessed in this stage; this stage also begins the assessment of the faculty and their perspectives, as well as the organization's goals. The second stage is the planning stage. During this stage, the faculty will be engaged and a topic will be decided upon. Other tasks will include choosing a speaker and preparing for the program delivery, as well as scheduling and evaluation needs. One likely question to ask in this stage is, "How will we organize the effort (support, deliver, schedule, and market the program)?" The next stage is the delivery stage. This is the stage of presenting the planned program. The final stage is follow-up. Evaluation of the program is accomplished during this stage. The educator will want to assess the meaning of the program to the individual and how to support the new learning within the organization.

Personal and professional development in students

It is important for students to take time out for reflection of what they have learned and understand how to apply it to their professional practice. Students should know what they are doing and understand why they are doing it. The student should never stop learning. As educators, it is important to remind our students of this fact. It is also important for educators and their peers to never stop learning, primarily through keeping abreast of the latest information by subscribing to or writing and researching for professional journals. Be involved with professional associations, in addition to attending conferences and further training. By performing these tasks, the educator can be a role model for students. Develop a personal development plan by asking such questions as; "What do I want to accomplish both personally and professionally?" and "What challenges do I see for myself?" By developing long-term goals, professional educators can develop their own personal mission and philosophy

Assessment and Evaluation Strategies

Validity of measurement tools

The current philosophy of validity does not focus on whether a test is valid for a specific purpose, nor on the tests themselves; instead, it focuses on the meaningfulness of the interpretation of the test scores. A particular test may be used for several different purposes, and as a result, test score results may have a greater validity for one purpose over another. Educators will need to determine the meaningfulness of the interpretations of test score results. These results can be utilized by instructors to make inferences about the test taker's knowledge and what he or she can do. The validity of the measurement tool will depend on to what extent these inferences are sound. For instructors to make good judgments about the validity of a set of test scores; they must gather one or more types of validity evidence. This validity evidence should include some or all of the following: criterion-related evaluations, content, and constructs.

Practicality of testing instruments

A testing instrument will be considered practical if it is fairly easy to administer, has reasonable resource requirements, and does not subtract too much time from instructional activities. Specific questions should be addressed when assessing the practicality of a measurement tool:
- Is the test easy to construct and use?
- Is the time needed to administer, score the test and interpret results reasonable?
- Are the costs associated with test construction, administration, and scoring reasonable?
- Can the test results be interpreted easily and accurately by those who will use them?"

Certain considerations must be taken into account when determining the practicality of a measurement tool. For example, an essay test may be easy to construct, but more difficult and time-consuming to grade. Students may achieve instructional goals during time spent in test preparation, but it is not the most effective way to achieve those instructional goals. Likewise, teacher-constructed tests may be less costly than published instruments, but the cost of the instructor's time must be considered.

Formative evaluations

Formative evaluation consists of the feedback to nursing students regarding their progress in meeting specific objectives and their competencies for practice. It occurs continuously throughout formal instruction, and will identify areas where further learning is needed. The instructor may use various methods in the classroom setting to perform formative evaluation. These methods can include small group activities, diagnostic quizzes, observation and questioning, and various written assignments. Formative evaluation is invaluable in assessing the nursing student's practice in the clinical setting. It will guide the nursing student's awareness of areas where performance may need to be improved. Since the main purpose of formative evaluation is to provide feedback to the instructor regarding a student's progress, it is not usually graded. By performing effective formative evaluation, the educator will be able to assess where more learning is needed.

Summative evaluations

Summative evaluation is used to determine what has been learned by the nursing student at the end of a course of study or clinical experience. It will demonstrate to what extent the course objectives have been achieved, and are utilized as a basis for grading the student. It will typically assess a broader area to be evaluated than formative evaluation. Some common methods used to perform summative evaluation include term papers, midterm or final exams, and other formal tests. Summative evaluation can be utilized in the nurse clinical setting as well. Some methods used to perform a summative evaluation of clinical skills include written assignments, portfolios, and completed clinical experience projects.

Cognitive domain learning

In order to properly assess and evaluate the nursing student's learning in the cognitive domain, objectives will need to be written which reflect the learning that is desired. Cognitive domain learning involves the acquisition of specific knowledge and facts, meaning the nursing student will need to develop an understanding of the theories and principles of nursing. Nursing students will demonstrate the ability to make decisions, problem-solve, and perform other types of critical thinking exercises. By writing specific objectives within the cognitive domain, the instructor will be able to plan instruction and carry out evaluation more appropriately. Objectives will need to be written which reflect the six levels of cognitive learning. These levels are knowledge, comprehension, application, analysis, synthesis, and evaluation.

Psychomotor domain learning

In order to properly assess and evaluate the nursing student's learning in the psychomotor domain, objectives will need to be written which reflect the type of learning that is desired. Psychomotor domain learning involves the acquisition of motor skills, which are based on what has been learned in the cognitive and the affective domains.

Psychomotor domain learning involves the development of competency and skills in the use of technology. Evaluation of this type of learning is usually performed in the clinical setting or learning laboratory. By writing specific objectives in the psychomotor domain, the instructor will be able to plan instruction and carry out evaluation more appropriately. Objectives will need to be written which reflect the five levels of psychomotor learning. These levels are imitation, manipulation, precision, articulation, and naturalization.

Affective domain learning

In order to assess and evaluate the nursing student's learning in the affective domain, objectives will need to be written which reflect the type of learning that is desired. Affective domain learning involves the development of beliefs, values, and attitudes which are consistent with professional nursing practice standards. Instruction goals should provide the student with assistance in developing a value system which reflects the core values of the nursing profession. This value system should guide students' decisions and behaviors in future practice. This type of learning is usually more difficult to evaluate, especially in the higher levels of affective domain learning. It involves the observation of nursing student behavior to determine if there is a commitment to act according to the taught professional values. By writing specific objectives in the affective domain, the instructor will be able to plan instruction and carry out evaluation more appropriately. Objectives will need to be written which reflect the five levels of affective learning, which are receiving, responding, valuing, organization, and characterization.

Expected outcomes of clinical practice

The following educational outcomes of clinical practice are expected of professional accredited nursing programs:
- Acquire concepts, theories, and other knowledge for clinical practice.
- Use research and other evidence for clinical decision making and evidence-based nursing practice.
- Use critical thinking skills in clinical practice.
- Develop psychomotor and technological skills and competence in other types of interventions.
- Develop professional values and knowledge essential to providing health care to a diverse and multicultural client population.
- Communicate effectively with patients and others in the health care system.
- Demonstrate leadership skills and behaviors of a professional nursing provider.
- Accept responsibility for actions and decisions.
- Accept need for continued learning and self development.

Clinical evaluations

Types

Educators should be aware that their own values will influence their clinical evaluation of their students. Judgments that instructors make about their students' performances will be made based on their own inherent values. It is important to keep this in mind so evaluations will be fair. Observations regarding a nursing student's performance will need to be compared to a set of standards to arrive at a fair evaluation. A criterion-referenced clinical evaluation involves comparing the student's clinical performance to a pre-determined set of criteria. A norm-referenced evaluation is when the student's clinical performance is measured against the performance of other students. Formative clinical evaluation provides feedback to the student to assist them in understanding their strengths and weaknesses. It moves the student forward in their learning by improving performance. Summative evaluation is done at the end of a clinical course to show whether clinical outcomes have been achieved. Confirmative evaluation shows if a student has maintained his or her competencies over time.

Feedback

When the educator provides feedback to the nursing student, it is important to be specific and provide an exact description about what is lacking. General statements about the student's behavior should be avoided. The student needs to know exactly where to focus efforts toward improvement. When a psychomotor skill is evaluated, it is helpful for the educator to provide both verbal and visual feedback. The teacher should explain verbally first, and then demonstrate the proper skill or procedure. Feedback should be timely; preferably, it should be given immediately at the time of learning or directly following it. Different students may need different amounts of feedback and positive reinforcement. Beginning students will usually require more. As time goes on, the more experienced student is capable of self-evaluation and becomes more confident so needs less positive reinforcement. There may also be a difference based on personalities of the students. The feedback process should be cyclical in nature. The educator first observes and evaluates, then gives feedback. Finally, the teacher guides the student into becoming more competent.

Selection of methods

Many different types of clinical evaluation methods are available to choose from when assessing the achievement of clinical outcomes. The instructor will need to review the expected outcomes of the course, and decide which method best measures the competency achieved. Often, one method may measure more than one outcome. Methods of assessment should be varied to maintain students' interest and allow for their differences, as some students are more proficient in one method over another. Methods should be realistic, given the amount of students to be evaluated and the required resources and expenses to evaluate them. Methods can be used for formative or summative evaluation, but the students should know how they are being used beforehand. A realistic number of assignments to achieve evaluation should be given. Students do not benefit from repetitive assignments that do not contribute to their development. When planning evaluation, the educator should consider the demands that will be placed on the time and effort of the nursing faculty.

Observation

The clinical competencies or outcomes will guide the educator in their observations. It is important to share all observations with the student to obtain input regarding the perceptions of their behaviors or actions. The instructor should keep in mind that observations can be biased, due to their own judgments and limitations or focus while observing. Several methods are used to record student observations, including anecdotal notes, checklists, and rating scales. Anecdotal notes are narrative descriptions written based on observations in the clinical setting. These notes should be recorded as close to the time of observation as possible. Checklists delineate steps expected to be accomplished when performing a particular skill. The instructor will identify how well and whether all were performed. This method allows the student to objectively view their performance. Rating scales are usually used in the summative evaluation stage. These scales include a list of outcomes and a judgment about how they were performed.

Simulation

Simulation is advantageous for nursing students, in that they can practice necessary skills without the constraints of a real-life situation. The simulator can offer changing situations, allowing the students to feel more comfortable practicing their reactions without the fear of harming a patient. Different types of simulations can be utilized for clinical evaluation. Case scenarios, interactive video, human patient simulators, CD-ROMs, and models or mannequins can all be useful in assessing clinical outcomes and competencies. Simulation laboratories can be equipped like an examination room or hospital room. To facilitate instructor evaluation, two-way mirrors, video cameras, microphones and other media can be utilized. Videoconferencing can also be utilized in the clinical setting. Standardized patients or actors are used as simulators. This allows for two way communication, and can be helpful in evaluating the communication techniques of the student. An OSCE, or Objective Structured Clinical Examination, is a means for evaluating in a simulation laboratory. All these simulation methods can be utilized for formative and/or summative evaluation.

Written assignments

Written assignments can be an effective method of evaluating the nursing student's problem-solving, critical thinking, and higher-level learning skills. They are most valuable in evaluating the achievement of clinical outcomes in Web-based and other distance education courses. Prompt feedback should be provided by the educator after reviewing the written assignment. By maintaining a journal, the nursing student can provide ongoing information in regards to his or her learning. This allows for formative evaluation by the instructor. Nursing care plans are another form of utilizing written assignments in clinical evaluation. The plans encourage the student's use of the nursing process, as well as further review of other learning resources. Concept maps are another form of written assignment. They are useful in helping the student understand the relationship between different sets of clinical data. They are an excellent visualization tool to assist the student in seeing how assessment data, diagnoses, and interventions relate. Other written evaluation assignments may include process recording, papers, and case studies.

<u>Conferencing</u>
Conferences are an excellent method used to evaluate the achievement of outcomes in the clinical setting. Several different types of conferences can be utilized. Pre-clinical conferences will be performed prior to the clinical experience. The educator can assess the students' knowledge and provide appropriate feedback prior to the clinical experience to enhance achievement of the learning objectives. Post-clinical conferences are held immediately following the clinical experience. Some possible tasks to accomplish during post-clinical conferences would be: collaboration with peers, assessing the effectiveness of interventions, and examining ethical dilemmas encountered. The educator can evaluate the students' ability to think critically and use the concepts and theories they have been taught. Conferences are usually evaluated for formative purposes.

<u>Distance education students</u>
When evaluating psychomotor and other clinical skills in the distance education student, observation and rating of performance are the most effective methods used. Observations can be performed by faculty onsite or distanced by the use of simulators, standardized patients, and other virtual reality devices. Checklists and rating scales can be used after reviewing the clinical performance onsite or through videoconferencing or videotaping. Clinical evaluation of cognitive outcomes and skills can be accomplished by using various written assignments. Such assignments might include electronic journals, short assignments for building critical thinking skills, term papers, or nursing care plans. Other forms of cognitive outcome and skill evaluation might include case presentations, online conferences and discussions, a student portfolio, and written testing.

Grading

In order to accurately reflect student achievement, grades should be provided after careful evaluation practices, reliable test results, and a variety of evaluation methods. Grades serve instructional, administrative and guidance, and counseling purposes.

Instructionally, grades measure what the student has learned and their achieved competencies. Grades also serve an administrative purpose, in that they can be used to determine admission to entry-level and higher degree nursing programs. Grades are used to determine the student's eligibility to graduate, or decisions about re-entry or probation in a nursing program. Grades are also useful in awarding scholarships, fellowships, honors or acceptance in honor societies, as well as being utilized in nursing program evaluation, and may be reported to employers. Finally, grades are useful in making decisions about courses to select, and whether remedial courses or other types of educational support are needed.

Principles of good practice

The principles of good practice for assessing students are as follows:
- Assessment is most effective when it reflects an understanding of learning as multidimensional, integrated, and revealed in performance over time.
- Assessment works best when the programs it seeks to improve have clear, explicitly stated purposes. Assessment is a goal-oriented process.
- Assessment requires attention to outcomes, but also and equally to the experiences that lead to those outcomes.
- Assessment works best when it is ongoing, not episodic.
- Assessment fosters wider improvement when representatives from across the educational community are involved.
- Assessment makes a difference when it begins with issues of use and illuminates questions that people really care about.
- Assessment is most likely to lead to improvement when it is part of a larger set of conditions that promote change.
- Through assessment, educators meet responsibilities to students and to the public.
- The assessment of student learning begins with educational values.

Changes in undergraduate nursing education programs

Changes are occurring in the traditional undergraduate nursing education programs. The nursing curricula and clinical education are being revitalized and restructured in order to adapt and survive in the future. A variety of nursing programs are being offered now to would-be nurses. Entrepreneurial organizations and traditional educational organizations are now offering LVN/LPN-to-RN programs or generic baccalaureate and associate degrees. There is a nursing shortage driving the need for licensed RNs to be developed quickly for the lowest cost, in order to provide much-needed bedside nurses. Technology has been another driving force of this type of education. Education can now be provided through virtual universities, and clinical practice can be obtained in simulation laboratories or virtual intensive care units. Opinions differ among nurse educators on which type of education is best. Concern exists regarding the credibility of a nontraditional versus a traditional nursing education program. Other causes of change from the traditional approach include shifting demographics and the knowledge explosion.

Evaluation focus

The most important step in planning an evaluation is to determine its focus. This will ultimately guide the design of the evaluation, how to conduct it, and how to analyze the data obtained, as well as the reporting of the results. The five basic components of the evaluation's focus are audience, purpose, questions, scope, and resources. The audience will usually include the individual or group who requested the evaluation. The purpose is basically why the evaluation is being conducted. For an evaluation to fulfill its purpose, the right questions must be asked. The scope includes what and how much is to be evaluated. It can basically be considered an answer to the question or questions that are asked. In order to have a successful evaluation, a realistic appraisal of the resources that are available should be made. Resources might include materials, equipment, available facilities, expertise, personnel, and time required.

Evaluation and assessment

Assessment is the process of gathering, summarizing, analyzing, and using data to ultimately act in a specific way or direction. Conversely, evaluation is the process of gathering, summarizing, analyzing, and using data to determine if that action was indeed successful. The purpose and timing of evaluation and assessment differ. It is important to note that assessment is performed prior to the program's start in order to determine the student's needs. Evaluation, on the other hand, needs to be performed periodically during the program to determine if the student's needs are being met. It should also be performed at the completion of the program to determine if all the needs were met and to what extent they were met. Assessment and evaluation planning should be performed together prior to the planning and initiation of the program.

Barriers to evaluation

Barriers to evaluation are generally classified in three main categories, which are lack of clarity, lack of ability, and fear of punishment or loss of self-esteem. Poorly defined evaluation focus produces a lack of clarity; the purpose must be understood before it will be successfully accomplished. It is important to state what decisions will be made as a result of the evaluation, and to identify the five components of evaluation focus: audience, purpose, questions, scope and resources. If there is a lack of resources or of knowledge of what resources are necessary; it will become a barrier. A remedy for lack of knowledge would be to consult or collaborate with experts in the field. Some resources that might be lacking are time and money. If evaluation is perceived as a judgment of the audience's personal worth, fear will result and become a barrier. The evaluator must realize the likely existence of fear, value the person more than the results, recognize achievements, and encourage efforts.

Analysis and interpretation of data

The way data will be analyzed will depend on the nature of the data and the focus of the evaluation. To analyze quantitative data, it will need to be organized and summarized. Statistics methods, such as frequency and percentages, will need to be utilized to help analyze the data. It will be important to select appropriate statistical procedures to interpret the type of data collected. The results should answer questions which were developed and addressed in the planning stages of the evaluation. Decisions about how the data will be analyzed will be made on the basis of the nature of the data gathered and by the evaluation's focus. It may be necessary to consult with an experienced data analyst when interpreting complex data and results. Not all data collected is complex; the complexity of data will depend on whether it is quantitative or qualitative.

Evaluation process

The educator will conduct an evaluation by utilizing the chosen instruments according to the methods selected for their implementation. An evaluation will be more successful if it is carefully planned. There are three specific methods which might be helpful in performing a successful evaluation. It may prove helpful to perform a pilot test first, which can be performed with a few individuals who are similar to the larger group. By performing a pilot test, potential problems with the evaluation procedure or results can be realized. This is essential when the evaluation is expensive, time-consuming, or the measuring instruments are newly developed. The second method is to include extra time for unexpected delays. Finally, it is helpful to maintain a sense of humor, especially when results are unexpected and not viewed as favorable to the audience.

Reporting evaluation results

It is important to report the results of an evaluation. Evaluations may be performed, but their results may never be shared with the focused audience. It is important to keep in mind certain guidelines when performing an evaluation, so that the results will more likely be reported to the appropriate audience. These guidelines will cause usable results to be reported in a timely fashion. It is important to keep in mind your audience, and present the results of the evaluation in a language they can use and that will be applicable to them. The evaluator should present these results in person if at all possible. When reporting results, the evaluator should address the purpose of the evaluation and answer the focused questions. An evaluator's report should not interpret data which was not collected, and an explanation of the limitations of data received should be provided. The educator should not make a conceptual leap to make conclusions which are not supported by the collected data.

Selection of evaluation method

The evaluation's focus will help determine the best evaluation design structure. The design structure of the evaluation will help determine the best methods to utilize. Evaluation methods are tools used to assist in data collection and the analysis of that data. The evaluator must decide what types of data are to be collected, and where the data will need to be taken from. It must be decided who will collect the data and how, when, and where it will be collected. Next, there should be a search of the literature to study similar evaluations which have been accomplished. Instruments which have been used frequently are more likely to have been thoroughly tested for validity and reliability. The identified instruments should be evaluated as to which ones would be most appropriate for the projected evaluation. They should have evidence of their reliability and validity when applying them to a similar population group. The instruments should be affordable, and should not require extensive training by personnel who are conducting the evaluation.

Roberta Straessle Abruzzese evaluation model

This model was first developed in 1978 to assist with the evaluation of staff development education. It assists in categorizing, conceptualizing, or classifying educational evaluation, and may be utilized for both staff and patient education. It provides a picture of how the five basic types of evaluation—process, content, outcome, impact, and program—relate to one another. It is pictorially represented in a pyramid shape, with the lowest amount of time and cost and the most frequently used evaluation types represented in the base of the pyramid. The most complex of the evaluation types, which is impact evaluation, is at the peak. This type of evaluation requires the greatest amount of time and cost, and is used with the least frequency.

Important terms

Career ladder concept: The concept that the nurse or educator can enter nursing practice or academia at a certain basic level of education, and continue along at particular steps or levels. In some educational programs, credit may be given towards a degree simply based on the nurse's experience and course work which has been already completed.
Concept-mapping: The interconnections and relationships between concepts and data represented in a graphic demonstration, in order to show the students' thinking processes.
Evaluation: The demonstration of the value of a program, product, procedure, objective, teaching method or performance of a student. It includes obtaining information for use in judging the worth of the above-listed items, or the potential for utilizing other approaches to attain specific objectives or goals.
Goal-based evaluation: This is an evaluation which is based on the stated goals of the particular subject being analyzed. It is often used in education. This evaluation is

dependent on the goals, purpose, and learning objectives of the program or curriculum.

Reflective practice: The continuous and self-regulated process which directs one's understanding and learning. It is the process of contemplating one's own experiences in applying knowledge to the practice of nursing under the direction of a nursing instructor. Reflective practice, applied to the nursing educator, involves reviewing and analyzing one's own teaching methods and determining what has worked well for their students.

Assessment: The process of collecting specific data about students to determine the importance and value of their needs, problems, and strengths in order to decide a direction for action, in order to facilitate the learning process.

SAM (Suitability Assessment of Materials): This is an instrument designed to measure the appropriateness of printed materials, illustrations, and videotaped or audio-taped instructions for patients in a particular population group. It includes 22 factors which are assessed. Some of these include literacy demand, graphics, layout and typography, and cultural appropriateness.

TOFHLA (Test of Functional Health Literacy in Adults): An instrument developed in the 1990s which is used to measure a patient's literacy level, using actual realistic documents from the hospital—such as drug labels, informed consent documents, and appointment slips—to determine a patient's reading and numeracy skills. It consists of two parts, which are reading comprehension and literacy. It is also available in a Spanish version.

Formative evaluation: This is a methodical and ongoing assessment of the success of the teaching process made throughout the program. It is used to manage, guarantee, or improve the quality of performance in the delivery of an educational program.

Summative evaluation: This is the methodical assessment of the degree to which individuals have learned the material taught, or the degree to which the objectives have been met as a result of the educational intervention.

Impact evaluation: This is the process of analyzing outcomes or effects of an educational activity. The process extends beyond the activity itself to address organizational and/ or societal effects which occur as a result.

Instructional objectives: These are the intended outcomes of the educational process. The objectives are written in reference to a particular aspect of a program or a total program of study. The objectives are content-oriented and teacher-centered. Instructional objectives are also referred to as educational objectives.

Curriculum Design

Guidelines for initiating curriculum development

Upon joining a particular nursing school, it is important for the educator to first become familiarized with the curriculum's mission, goals, philosophy, and organizing structure or framework. The educator should continue to monitor the soundness of the curriculum on an ongoing basis. The educator should guarantee the degree of excellence of the nursing education provided by the institution by assessing the elements, processes, and outcomes of the curriculum. The faculty should include practicing nurses and other health care providers in curriculum planning sessions, in order to obtain up-to-date information on current and future health care trends. It is crucial that educators keep abreast of changes, advances in health care information, and new information by utilizing technology through computers, research, and the Internet. Students should be included in the process of curriculum evaluation to ascertain the success of achieving the program outcomes.

Responsibilities of performing curriculum development

When developing a curriculum, nursing faculty should ensure that the following responsibilities are met:
- Nursing faculty should produce policies and procedures which influence the behavior of nursing students and the faculty, as well as the curriculum.
- Faculty should act as advisors on educational issues.
- Faculty should oversee the content and learning experiences, so that they are in a logical order and progression to achieve learning objectives or outcomes.
- Faculty should be instrumental in collecting and analyzing pertinent information needed for the development of the curriculum and its revision when needed.
- Faculty should assist in preparing nursing students to be able to operate in a health care environment which is constantly changing and becoming more complex.
- Nursing faculty should facilitate idea sharing and strategize with regard to decision making, and the revision and development of curriculum.

Lancaster's formula for collaborative research

The six Cs of Lancaster's (1985) formula for collaborative research is commitment, compatibility, communication, contribution, consensus, and credit.

Commitment is the requirement of the institution to donate and commit certain resources needed in order to develop the curriculum. These resources might include time, space needed to meet and conduct research, finances, and the professionals for the committee. Compatibility refers to the need for the members to work well together as a team to meet a mutual goal. To enhance communication (the third C), subcommittees may be formed to save time in discussion. A gatekeeper may also be utilized to ensure the chance of each group member to express their ideas and be heard. In this way, each group member will be given an opportunity to contribute (the fourth C). Members of the curriculum development committee should mutually come to a majority agreement on the curriculum, which represents the fifth C, consensus. Finally, every member should be given credit, the sixth C, for their contributions.

Issues that impact curriculum development

In order to develop an appropriate curriculum, faculty must be aware of national/global health care trends and the needed skills or competencies required to meet these needs. There is more nursing education being provided by means of distance education technology, thus requiring educators to develop a curriculum that will be appropriate for this type of educational vehicle. Some nursing instructors may not feel comfortable or skilled in developing this type of curriculum. A supportive administration will be needed to assist instructors in developing the skills they will need to meet this demand. Certain demographic trends will also need to be considered during curriculum development; for example, there are increasing numbers of elderly and ethnically diverse patient populations. Environmental issues will also impact curriculum development. Some issues to consider include the threat of bioterrorism and multiple sources of pollution. Community-based nursing services are becoming a more essential part of the nursing curriculum. It is important for faculty to periodically review the curriculum and determine what is most essential and up-to-date.

Reflection of institution in curriculum design

The institution's philosophy and mission must be reflected in the curriculum. It is important for the faculty responsible for curriculum development to reach agreement with regard to how to best support and reflect the mission of the institution. The curriculum should support the institution and faculty's beliefs about education and people. Elements of a mission statement include the population which will be served; the geographic area served; the teaching, research and service goals of the institution; and the outcome desired for its nursing graduates. The faculty must identify the organization's philosophy and mission statement. Once this is identified and acknowledged, then the faculty will need to agree on how to contribute through the development of the curriculum. This will guide the faculty in identifying desired program outcomes and learning objectives.

Educational objectives in curriculum design

The educational objectives should be identified from information obtained through boards of nursing, community-needs assessment, accrediting agencies, and the concepts and ideals of educators involved in their development. In order to develop educational objectives, faculty must first identify the global objectives for the program. Global objectives are statements which reflect thoughtful, practical communication of the needs of the immediate community, both presently and in the future. Global goals are broader than instructional goals, and often will not reflect specific behaviors or outcomes. These global objectives should reflect a summary of the learning outcomes expected. Educational objectives should identify the kind of behavior to be developed and the content in which the behavior is to operate. These objectives should be written at three different levels. The first should address the general achievement expected over the course of a specific academic period of time. The next should address a class or unit within a course of study. The final level should address a specific lesson within a class or unit.

Cognitive domain knowledge types

The cognitive domain of learning encompasses intellectual skills, and includes four types of knowledge. Factual knowledge includes the basic information that students must be familiar with in order to solve problems within their discipline. The nursing student must know medical terminology, basic anatomy and physiology, and foundations of nursing. Conceptual knowledge is the process of defining interrelationships between the basic elements of factual knowledge. Nursing theories for understanding the health care system involve such conceptual knowledge. Procedural knowledge involves the skills of knowing how to perform a specific procedure, and the reasoning behind why it is performed. The nursing student must understand how and when it is necessary to utilize sterile technique, for example. Metacognitive knowledge involves the highest level within the cognitive domain. It is thinking with respect to an awareness of one's own thinking. This level involves the ability of the student to understand his or her own strengths and weaknesses and to take action to rectify those weaknesses.

Master plan of evaluation

Specific personnel should be identified who will collect data, analyze the findings, prepare the report of the findings, and distribute the information to these key people. A timeline should be established for collection, analysis, and the reporting of the identified pertinent data. A feedback loop should be in place to develop recommendations and for decisions to be made in response to the data obtained through evaluations. The master plan of evaluation findings should identify existing and potential problems, and should identify previously overlooked or new needs. Successes should be acknowledged and evaluated as to why they were successful. There should be advisement regarding improvements to be made, new programs to be started, or whether the program should be discontinued. Finally, there should be a plan made to implement these changes which delineates timelines and people responsible to accomplish them.

Challenges facing future curricula

There are several challenges that will affect the development of nursing curricula in the future. There will continue to be a nursing shortage, due to the expected increased demand for nurses in relation to the projected growth of the supply of nurses. The fastest growing segment of the nursing workforce is in community health settings. Hospitals continue to keep in-patient hospital stays to a minimum. Patients in the hospitals are in need of greater acute care. All of these changes have occurred rapidly, which creates a burden to rapidly change nursing curricula in order to meet the needs of appropriate nursing education. A challenge of the future is to coordinate care between the acute and less-acute, or community health, setting. It is a challenge to prepare nurses to function in both of these settings adequately. Nurses will require greater case management skills and supervisory skills, due to the expected increase of ancillary personnel to supplement the shortage of nurses.

There are numerous implications which can be identified to address the challenges that will face the development of nursing curricula. There will be an increased need for advanced-practice nurses, case managers, nursing administrators, and staff nurses who specialize in the care of the elderly. Nurses must be prepared by their educational institutions to function across all settings. They must be trained to function well in the community health, as well as the acute care, setting. They must understand how to coordinate services between both settings. It is essential to develop internships for nurses in order for them to obtain the necessary experience they need to function in both settings. They must be able to apply the educational knowledge to actual, realistic experience. The internship or residency would be instrumental in promoting critical thinking skills, clinical skills, and the transition to a professional nursing role.

Recommendations from The Institute of Medicine

The Institute of Medicine made several recommendations for health care professionals with regard to their educational preparation. One recommendation for education is to prepare the nurse to provide patient-centered care, which means the nurse must be prepared to work as part of an interdisciplinary team. The nurse should also be prepared to practice evidence-based medicine. This would involve utilizing the best evidence available in making decisions about patient or client care. The nurse should keep focused on the quality improvement of care. The nurse should be adept at using information technology. The Institute of Medicine recommends that specific professional entities should be responsible for ensuring that health professional education curricula includes all of the above recommended content. These entities might encompass certification organizations, as well as accreditation and licensing agencies.

Goal-based and goal-free evaluation

Goal-based evaluation is an evaluation of a program based on the stated goals of that program. The evaluation will be made based on the success of meeting the stated goals, the purpose, and the course objectives of the curriculum. Goal-free evaluation is a method used when evaluating a program without prior knowledge of its curriculum or its stated goals or purpose. The program is assessed and judged based entirely on the program itself, and not on whether it met its particular goals. The evaluator is an expert in the field of study being evaluated, and should have no prior knowledge of the program; this will produce a more bias-free evaluation. Goal-free evaluation will examine the actual effects of the program. These effects may include the actual intended effects as well as unintended effects. There may also be side effects and secondary effects which occur due to the program being evaluated.

Technology

Utilization for health care consumer
The World Wide Web is a wonderful health education resource for both the patient or client and the health care professional. Search engines, such as Google or Yahoo!, are vital resources for the information seeker so that a particular subject can be researched on the Web. The Internet allows an exchange of information between a global network of computers making knowledge of these technology resources essential for nurses working with the health care client. In order for the World Wide Web to be utilized to enhance the nurse educator's development of curriculum, the educator needs to be wise to its potential as a huge resource to the typical health care consumer. The nurse educator will require information literacy skills to ascertain the accuracy of the information obtained. It is important for the nurse educator to be prepared to share and develop this skill in the health care consumer as well.

The nurse educator can assist the health care consumer to feel at ease in sharing the information they may have gathered through the use of technology. The client should feel that the nurse educator is interested in discussing the information they have gathered in a nonjudgmental way. It is important for the nurse to review with the client the sites they have visited if at all possible with computer access available during the session. This will enable the nurse to assess the type and amount of information, the client's knowledge of it, and areas where further instruction may be necessary. Information clients have gathered that seems to conflict with what they have been taught will need to be addressed. Further instruction may be necessary to clear up misconceptions and discrepancies.

Information literacy

The information-literate individual should be able to identify the specific information they are seeking. The questions they are seeking answers for will need to be identified. The individual should have an understanding and ability to access the needed information. The information that is recovered must be evaluated by the individual intelligently for its accuracy and trustworthiness. Once the information is determined to be valid, it should be accurately utilized by the individual to meet their needs.

An individual who is computer-literate may have the technical skills and an understanding of the technology, but may be unable to evaluate the accuracy of the information obtained through computer usage.

Teaching tool

The professional nurse educator needs to be aware of and familiar with the research that has been conducted on the effects of distance education technologies and student outcomes. Thomas Russell performed a study which revealed that there is a lack of evidence to support a difference in student outcome between students educated traditionally versus those who received a technology-based education. Technology is increasing and advancing at an extremely rapid pace. It is difficult for the educator to keep up with all the new information and technology-based strategies that are being developed on a daily basis. There is now a growing body of research on the use of technology as a teaching tool for patient education as well. Most of these studies are smaller in scope than that performed by Russell. The professional educator must view technology as a vehicle to deliver programs and promote learning. Technology is a powerful tool, which must be used thoughtfully and cautiously in education.

Support for older population

Research has revealed that the older segment of the population is one of the groups that may not have the resources necessary to access technology. Research has shown that as a group, more than half of Americans between the ages of 60-69 actually have Internet access, but the use of it diminishes with increasing age. However, research has demonstrated that with education and support, these same adults enjoy learning from technology-based educational programs.

The nurse educator can help this population group by assisting in trouble-shooting ergonomic limitations in the elderly. Education regarding proper posture and correct positioning of the keyboard is one example of support. For those with limited access, the educator can provide a list of free computer access resources and places where seniors can obtain free technology training. Providing a supportive, nonthreatening environment for learning and helping seniors identify with how the technology can meet their personal needs.

Core competencies and competency statements

Core competency is an area of expertise in a specific subject area or skill set. Core competencies comprise the essential knowledge, skills, and attitudes necessary for practice. Core competencies also relate to the practice of individuals. They can serve as a tool for assessing and creating the best mix of competency statements for a specific role or educational goal.

Competency statements are a description of the behavior that is expected from the student. A competency can consist of a range of skills, knowledge, and attitudes. It must be described as a measurable or observable action. All competency statements should include a verb and its object, or observable or measurable action. A broad competency statement would describe the behavior that is expected from an individual acting in a particular role or position. A narrow competency statement would describe the observable behavior that is expected or anticipated upon course completion or mastery of a particular skill or group of skills.

Identifying appropriate program outcomes

The overall purpose of a program is influenced by the type of nursing education it is intended to deliver. The program outcomes will differ between the different types of programs. The different nursing education programs include licensed practical or vocational nurse, associate, baccalaureate, and masters or doctoral degree preparation. The overall purpose or goal of a program will act as a guide in developing end-of-program objectives or outcomes. In order to develop or identify program outcomes, the educator must analyze the program's mission, purpose, and overall goal. The program outcomes will serve as a master plan for determining what content should be included in the curriculum.

Philosophy statement

A statement of philosophy is developed to flow from the mission statement of an institution of higher learning. Faculty members who develop this statement must create a general philosophical statement based on their own personal philosophies. The statement should reflect the rationale for the nursing school's existence. This statement will be instrumental in guiding curriculum development. The essential components of a philosophical statement should reflect the faculty's consensus on their values, beliefs, attitudes about nursing, and how to impart the knowledge of nursing to students. Components of the philosophy include statements on theories of learning and teaching, how to incorporate critical thinking skills in learning, how to impart knowledge to the diverse student, and the inclusion of the nursing metaparadigm.

The philosophy must be in agreement with what is currently or expected to be taught in the immediate future. If a lack of congruence begins to develop, then it may be time to change or revise the philosophy statement.

Evaluation of educational programs

Tyler Model

The Tyler Model is also called the "objectives model" or "goal attainment model." It is based on four main principles. The first principle is to define the appropriate learning objectives of the program. Learning experiences which are useful must then be established. These learning experiences should be organized in a way to bring about the greatest cumulative effect. Finally, the curriculum should be evaluated and those aspects which were ineffective should be revised. By utilizing this evaluation model, the nurse educator can take action to eliminate programs or components of the curriculum which do not contribute to quality outcomes.

CIPP model

The CIPP (Context, Input, Process, and Product) evaluation model is based on the viewpoint that evaluation findings should be used to improve the program, not to prove the program. The *context evaluation* identifies the strengths and weaknesses of the nursing education program, and enhances curriculum revision with the information obtained. The *input evaluation* will help determine what approach should be taken to bring about the change that is needed. During this phase of the evaluation, a comparison of the program being evaluated to existing programs elsewhere may prove helpful. The *process evaluation* involves the evaluator gathering information in an unobtrusive manner in order to ascertain whether the curriculum is on track. In this way, changes can be made during the program's course so that the objectives of the program will more likely be met. The *product evaluation* involves obtaining feedback from stakeholders in the program. Stakeholders are members of the group that the program is intended to serve. The stakeholders will provide feedback on whether their educational needs were met by the program.

Curriculum in client-centered health education and schools of nursing

Many of the same elements of curriculum development and evaluation in schools of nursing apply to its development in a client-centered health education and staff development arena. A needs assessment will still need to be performed to determine the needs of the identified student. Just as the mission, goals, and philosophy of a nursing education program must be in agreement with its sponsoring institution; the mission, goals, and philosophy of the health education program and staff development program must be in line with the sponsoring health agency's mission, goals, and philosophy. The same program evaluation theories, models, and concepts can be applied to assess the outcomes of the client-centered health education and staff development programs.

Critical thinking

Goals for education

The first goal is to defend, promote, and articulate elevated standards of research, scholarship, and teaching in critical thinking. The second goal is to communicate the criteria upon which quality thinking is based, as well as the standards of which this thinking can be assessed and grown. The third goal involves assessing the programs that strive to provide such higher-order critical thinking. The final goal is to distribute information which assists educators as well as others in identifying programs and various approaches which provide quality critical thinking within their curriculum. This will help to reform and restructure education systematically in order to cultivate disciplined universal and intellectual standards within specific domains.

Principles

The following is an overview of the first seven principles of critical thinking as established by the National Council for Excellence in Critical Thinking:

1. Knowledge and thinking are intimately interrelated.
2. Knowing that something is true is not just a matter of "knowing," but being justified in the belief that it is true.
3. The assessment of thinking encompasses general as well as domain-specific standards.
4. It is essential to think critically in order to truly achieve knowledge within any domain.
5. Since critical thinking is based on specific intellectual standards, it must also be assessed by those same standards.
6. There are certain standards that have historically been essential to the assessment of one's thinking within all domains. Some of these general standards include accuracy, fairness, logic, relevance, significance, probability, and evidentiary support.
7. Teaching in critical thinking should lead students to exhibit some of the above mentioned standards, so that they will practice a disciplining of the mind and commitment to apply these standards to a life of intellectual and moral integrity.

Learning activities

Some critical thinking activities that can be employed are concept mapping, debate on a subject, and writing-to-learn. In order to write-to-learn, the instructor must provide accurate, quality literature for the students to review. The educator should provide guidance to the students on how to organize the literature in a logical way, so that they can adequately write about their beliefs and values about the material. Some ways of incorporating writing-to-learn activities for the student are creative writing assignments, journal writing, or writing a summary of research with a position statement provided.

A concept mapping activity will require students to organize their thoughts and demonstrate this organization on paper in a graphic manner. A concept map provides a visual on how the material is related and interconnected. This activity expands the students' ability to assess their own thinking, and requires them to explain the connections and relationship they have demonstrated on paper. Debate requires much research and knowledge on the topic, and the ability to support evidence through logical argument and logical thinking.

Evaluation of outcomes or competencies

Clinical outcomes are sometimes expressed as clinical objectives. Sometimes, the outcomes are expressed more broadly by faculty. The faculty will then specify certain behaviors the students will exhibit, which will show they are meeting the outcomes in a chosen course of study. The outcomes or competencies must be stated in specific enough terms to guide the evaluation of students in clinical practice, and must be specific enough to be measured by a chosen evaluation tool or method. A nurse's competencies for practice are simply the proficiencies needed by the nurse in order to perform or carry out a particular task or skill. A realistic number of competencies or outcomes should be developed by the educator so that evaluation of them is possible within the time frame of the course and the amount of students served.

Program evaluation models

Several program evaluation models exist for use in nursing, staff, and patient education. The models assist educators in developing a plan for evaluation. Information for quality improvement is provided to educators when they perform a planned, well-organized evaluation. Some accreditation models are used by the National League for Nursing Accrediting Commission, the Commission on Collegiate Nursing Education, and Joint Commission on Accreditation of Healthcare Organizations (JCAHO). These agencies often use a combination of self-study and onsite visits by a peer evaluator team.

Another type of evaluation model is the decision-oriented model, which focuses more on internal standards of quality, merit, and the effect of the program. Some decision-oriented models are the CIPP model and the Baldridge Criteria. Systems-oriented models are another type of evaluation model, which examine the outcomes of the program.

Curriculum evaluation and program evaluation

Curriculum evaluation and program evaluation are not the same. Curriculum evaluation has a more narrow scope than program evaluation. The focus of curriculum evaluation is on the courses taken by the students, and whether the curriculum has been implemented as planned, among many other measures. Program evaluation has a broader scope; it not only includes all areas addressed by curriculum evaluation, but also looks at how the program relates to the institution. Other areas examined by program evaluation may include student support services, program resources, and a look at other aspects that influence its effectiveness. The success of the students meeting curriculum objectives or expected outcomes depends on many things that relate to the program's effectiveness, and thus its evaluation. For instance, the success of meeting objectives may depend on the effectiveness of the faculty and/or the quality of students that are admitted to the program.

Needs assessment

External frame factors

A needs assessment is the process of collecting and examining information which could influence the creation or revision of an educational program. Some common external frame factors which may influence the needs assessment are as follows. The community in which the program will exist and have an appeal must be studied and described. The financial viability of the program is assessed with regard to resources for scholarships and financial aid. The actual need for the program is assessed. The characteristics of the academic setting, the political climate, and demographics are taken into consideration. The potentially served health care systems and the health needs of the surrounding population are also assessed. A search of nursing professions in the region should be performed to determine available resources for financial aid, as well as educators and leaders or mentors. Finally, requirements of the regulating bodies or accreditation agencies must be reviewed.

Internal frame factors

Internal frame factors are factors which affect the educational program and the curriculum. These factors can impact decisions about changes in the program and the program's existence. One internal frame factor is the description and organizational structure of the parent academic institution. This description will include such things as how the nursing program fits within the political environment of the institution. It may also include where the program is located on campus, and what resources the institution provides for the program. The potential faculty and student characteristics comprise another internal frame factor which will affect the program. An example of this could be the available faculty to provide an appropriate student-faculty ratio. The parent institution's mission or purpose, philosophy, and goals make up another internal frame factor. Finally, the resources within the institution and nursing program, as well as the internal economic situation and its influence on the curriculum, will comprise other internal frame factors.

Curriculum revision

Some possible steps educators could take when revising their program's curriculum are:
- Identify the need for the revision to the curriculum through evaluation methods.
- Remember that every member of the faculty is involved in curriculum development.
- Appoint a committee to perform the needed revision.
- Remain focused on the committee's ultimate goals of revision, which should be in keeping with the overall program's goals.
- Resources to assist with the revision should be identified.
- Keep all faculty informed and involved with the revision process.
- Present proposed revisions and seek a buy-in from all faculty members. A consensus on the revision should be sought.

Important terms

Cocurriculum: This term is also referred to as informal curriculum. This term refers to activities that occur outside of the planned curriculum, but are still a part of the educational experience. These activities might include various ceremonies, athletic events, and club-related meetings.

Curriculum: This is a formalized plan of study developed by educators, administrators, and other experts in the specific field. It provides direction for the delivery of an educational program by identifying the goals of the program of study that are in agreement with its philosophy.

Curriculum evaluation: The process of evaluating a curriculum and its effectiveness. Decisions and judgments about a program of study can be made by gathering information about the curricula. By looking at the structure of a curriculum and analyzing it, the educator will be able to evaluate the program's effectiveness and value to achieving the goals of the program of study.

Philosophy: The study of global or universal complexities concerning matters such as one's existence, discovered information, what is truth, what is beauty, what is just, what is valid, etc. Philosophy uses a systematic approach to address these questions or subjects. The answers are provided through a reasoned argument. The word *philosophy* is derived from the ancient Greek word *philosophía*, which means "the love of wisdom."

Metaphysics: This branch of philosophy attempts to answer the questions of what is real and true. It is concerned with explaining the ultimate nature of existing, and how it relates to the world around us. It is intimately connected with epistemology.

Epistemology: This is a branch of philosophy which involves the study of nature, knowledge validity, and what is the difference between what is true and what is an opinion in relationship to human knowledge.

Axiology: This is a branch of philosophy which involves the study and description of what is ethical, aesthetical, logical, and of value.

Life-long learning

It is important for educators to take time out of teaching to reflect on their own personal development. Educators must understand why they are doing what they are doing (teaching), and what exactly they are doing or accomplishing. Stephen Covey provides a story in his literature about two lumberjacks, one who kept sawing wood because he wanted to not take time from his task, and the other who noticed his saw was getting dull and so decided to take time to sharpen it. In the end, the one who sharpened his saw cut more wood. The moral of the story is that professionals need to take time out of their everyday responsibilities to others to improve themselves or sharpen their own "saws." Students are becoming more technologically savvy, and knowledge is becoming more readily accessible through the Internet, so educators need to keep up-to-date on the latest research and technology if they are going to be effective educators.

There are many wonderful ways for the educator to continue life-long learning. It is important to join and participate in professional organizations. Professional networks and associations exist in many nursing specialties, and it is crucial that educators become familiar with the networks and associations within their specialty area. These professional organizations will also have periodicals, journals, and newsletters with the latest information in the field specialty. Often, these same organizations will offer conferences and other seminars to obtain continuing education. It is imperative for educators to develop their own personal development plan. This will provide them with a sense of direction and a plan for their own personal development in the future. Performing one's own professional research will grow an educator's knowledge of the most up-to-date information. Educators should enroll in applicable classes themselves to continue to grow in their knowledge and learning.

Committee work

It is not unusual for faculty members to be involved with several committees. These committees may be department-specific, or serve the institution as a whole. Faculty members may volunteer to serve on a committee, or they could be appointed to a committee. Committees will be different in nature. Some will not require a lot of time outside of their meetings, and may even meet infrequently. Other committees may be very time-intensive, and require a lot of work by the members on their own outside of the meeting times. Committee work involves participation in the duties of a deliberative assembly that is usually subordinate to a larger deliberative assembly. Committees serve several functions, which might include governance, coordination, research and recommendations, and project management.

FERPA

The nursing educator must be aware of the Family Educational Rights and Privacy Act (FERPA) of 1974, also known as the Buckley Amendment. This law requires students' records—which include grades, their attendance, health records and their academic standing—to remain private. Several other aspects of maintaining students' privacy need to be understood. Grades may not be shared with any other students, or even the students' parents, unless there is written permission to do so. In some institutions, if parents submit a federal income tax form which shows they support the student, they may have access. Grades may not be posted by name, Social Security number or any other identifiable way in order to maintain the students' privacy. Students may not deliver another student's grades to them. Student conferences should be held in the strictest confidence and privacy. This law also maintains that the student should have access to their academic record with advance notice.

Failing students

Faculty is required to provide students with *due process* in the event the student is failing. *Due process*, or more fully "due process of the law," is the principle that the government must respect all of the legal rights that are owed to someone according to the law of the land. In regards to the failing student, the educator should provide regular reports of the student's progress. Graded assignments must be returned in a timely manner, so the student is aware of his or her grade. It is important to provide written feedback, at the very least, at the midpoint of the course. If the student is failing, written feedback should be provided as frequently as possible, as this provides the student with fair warning that performance is not up to par. Another part of due process is to provide information regarding requirements at the beginning of the course, so students are aware of the passing standards. Students should also be given the opportunity to appeal their grade through a formal appeal process.

Academic dishonesty

Faculty is required to provide *due process* in the event that a student is suspected of or discovered performing in an academically dishonest manner. *Due process* of the law is the principle that the government must respect all of the legal rights that are owed to someone according to the law of the land. Academic dishonesty includes such activities as cheating, plagiarism, and lying. Before disciplinary action can be taken against a student accused of performing an academic dishonesty, they must be given due process. The student must also be given the right to appeal. There should be a formal appeal process in place at the institution for this purpose.

Tenure

Tenure, essentially the guarantee of employment except for extreme or unusual circumstances, is usually achieved after the new faculty member has completed a four- to six-year probationary period. New faculty members must complete this probationary period in order to "prove" themselves to the hiring institution. During this probationary period, new educators are expected to accomplish several professionally-related tasks. One of these tasks may include performing research, with publications and presentations as a result. Educators will need to provide effective service, and demonstrate the ability to get along with their professional colleagues. Institutions may vary on their tenure requirements and number of tenure positions. Once tenure is achieved, the faculty member may assume he or she will have the faculty position for life, unless the department is eliminated or there are definite grounds for dismissal.

Post-tenure review

Post-tenure review involves the periodic review of a tenured faculty member's accomplishments, and thus his or her effectiveness. A tenured faculty member's accomplishments are usually presented in a professional portfolio. These professional portfolios may include several types of documents which demonstrate the educator's accomplishments. These accomplishments help to provide an overall picture of faculty members, emphasizing their strengths. These strengths will help to enhance the educators' ability to be retained and/or promoted. Some documents which may be included in a portfolio include: a summary statement about teaching strengths, goals, and professional growth; samples of teaching materials and student work with their written feedback; peer and student evaluations; list and samples of publications or scholarship; and an updated curriculum vitae.

Faculty mentoring

Faculty mentoring means the provision of guidance and direction by more experienced faculty members to new or less experienced faculty members. Mentoring may include not only guiding new, inexperienced faculty members, but also experienced faculty members who are new to the institution or who are in need of adjusting their teaching techniques to an ever-changing health care environment or student population. Less experienced faculty members will require assistance in developing effective teaching skills with small and large groups. They will need support and guidance in grading activities. Experienced faculty members can provide assistance to the inexperienced educator in planning solid clinical experiences for students. The new educator will require assistance in adapting to the role as an academic advisor to their students. Experienced faculty members, though experienced in their teaching role, may require some mentoring and support with adapting to new information technologies in the constantly expanding and rapidly growing nursing education arena.

Reflective practice groups

Reflective practice is a type of evaluation that incorporates two elements. Reflection-in-action includes a self-evaluation while performing a particular practice activity, so that an improvement can be made immediately. Reflection-on-action involves more of a retrospective reflection on an activity after its completion. A reflective practice group for teachers would focus on the reflection-on-action element. This type of practice group is an important step in the support of a faculty member's learning and development. Organized, systematic reflection with colleagues will help nursing faculty better understand their assumptions, which ultimately lead to their beliefs and subsequently their actions. Monthly staff meetings can be an excellent time to accomplish peer reflective practice. By reflecting in an organized way about specific topics for discussion, alternative ways of thinking and behaving can be explored and envisioned.

Peer evaluation

Peer evaluation is the assessment of a professional educator's teaching effectiveness by his or her professional colleagues. There are numerous techniques used to accomplish this type of evaluation. One technique may involve the observation of the teacher in the classroom setting, laboratory, or clinical setting. Often this type of evaluation can be affected by the evaluator's personal feelings about his or her colleague, whether positive or negative. Web-based courses may also undergo peer evaluation. The evaluator may review course materials and visit the course Web site. Peer evaluators may review course syllabi, tests, grants, publications, and the teaching portfolio, as well as the observation of teaching strategies and learning activities.

Effectiveness in the clinical setting

In order to evaluate an instructor's effectiveness in the clinical teaching setting, there are some helpful questions that may be asked. Did the instructor facilitate learning in the clinical setting? Did the nursing instructor provide good feedback on students' strengths and weaknesses in relationship to their performance in the clinical setting? Did the educator develop positive relationships with his or her students? Did the teacher encourage and support student and health care team member cooperation to achieve learning? Was the teacher available to assist the students in the health care setting? Did the educator encourage inquisitiveness from his or her students and a feeling of acceptance to express differing views in the clinical setting?

Evaluation by students

Areas of assessment
There are several typical areas which are assessed by students when evaluating their instructors. Some of these areas include the teacher's presentation or teaching skills, interactions with students, coverage of the course material, and finally the evaluation and grading practices. When evaluating an instructor's presentation or teaching skills, some areas to assess may include the following:
- Were clear explanations provided?
- Was the course organized well, and was the instructor well-prepared for class?
- Did the educator motivate the students to do their best and stimulate their interest in the material?
- When evaluating interactions with their students, did the teacher encourage student participation and discussion?
- Was he or she available to the students?
- When evaluating the coverage of the material, did the instructor demonstrate knowledge and present different viewpoints?
- When evaluating grading practices, were the expectations clearly stated and evaluation methods explained?
- Was quick and appropriate feedback provided?

Effectiveness
There are several factors which may affect student evaluations of an instructor's effectiveness, thus making them an insufficient source of evaluation. Sometimes ratings or evaluations given by students may be affected by class size. The smaller the class size, the more effective the teacher may be perceived to be. The course format itself may affect a student's evaluation of the instructor. Discussion courses tend to have a higher rating of teacher effectiveness than a lecture format course. If students are taking a course in their own major or required course of study, the teacher may be rated as more effective, as opposed to an elective course. Students do not have the expertise to truly evaluate a teacher's knowledge of the subject matter, since they are just learning the subject themselves.

National League for Nursing

The National League for Nursing developed and provides the Certification for Nurse Educators (CNE). The NLN provides many opportunities for faculty development. One of these activities includes the annual Education Summit. The NLN sponsors and provides institutes and conferences on technology, curriculum development, and nursing education research. The NLN co-sponsors and helps to coordinate regional workshops on nursing education-related topics. It provides various audio/Web seminars and online courses. NLN is a provider for continuing education units through the International Association of Continuing Education and Training (IACET). The NLN Foundation for Nursing Education, along with the NLN, helps to empower nurse educators throughout America. By providing scholarships, grants, research, and faculty development programs, they endeavor to promote excellence in nursing education.

Publications
The National League for Nursing's mission is to advance excellence in nursing education. The publications provided by the NLN provide a broad range of resources to nursing educators. The NLN journal *Nursing Education Perspectives* provides articles which are peer-reviewed, and is published on a bimonthly basis. NLN publishes print and electronic newsletters which include *The NLN Report, NLN Member Update, Professional Development Bulletin,* and *Nursing Education Policy.* The NLN's Divisions of Research and Professional Development publish publications as well, some of which include *The Scope of Practice for Academic Nurse Educators* and the *National Study of Faculty Role Satisfaction.* Several books are available through the NLN as well to provide valuable information to nursing educators. Some of these books include (2008) Nursing Data Review; Academic Year 2005-2006; (2007) Nurse Educator Competencies: Creating an Evidence-Based Practice for Nurse Educators; and (2007) Simulation in Nursing Education: From Conceptualization to Evaluation.

World Wide Web

The World Wide Web provides numerous professional resources to nurse educators. There are many Web sites which have been developed by nursing organizations and publishing companies. These Web sites provide an abundance of information and services, which can answer all types of professional educator needs. The professional educator can access bibliographic databases, online journals, patient teaching and professional practice resources, and continuing education opportunities. Some examples of Web sites that may be utilized by nursing educators include Medline Plus (http://www.nln.nih.gov/medlineplus), Mayoclinic.com (http://www.mayohealth.org), Cancer Net (http://www.nci.hih.gov), NetWellness (http://www.netwellness.org), National Institutes of Health (http://www.nih.gov), and AllNursingSchools.com (http://www.allnursingschools.com).

It is important to note that e-learning provides learning opportunities at the point of need. Nursing educators must be just as current on the latest technology as the nursing workforce. The nursing workforce often is educated through the use of e-learning modalities in the workplace setting, so the nurse educator must be experienced in this method of learning as well, in order to communicate its importance to future nurses. Webcasts are another technological avenue to be utilized by educators to continue their life-long learning. Webcasts may include Webinars or Web conferencing. Webinars often have a computer-based display and a live discussion. Mobile learning, or m-learning, is another technological method utilizing wireless, portable, mobile, or handheld devices. Distance education is basically students studying at a distance. It may be delivered by many different methods, but is usually provided by computer through the use of the Internet and administered by an educator who is employed by an institution.

Nursing educator shortage

The National League for Nursing has identified a current and expected increase in the shortage of nurse educators. There is concern about the number of faculty who are available and adequately prepared for the role of nursing educators. Due to the overall nursing shortage in America, and the expected increased need due to the diverse and aging population, enrollment in nursing schools needs to be increased. The NLN states it is necessary to increase the enrollments by as much as one-third to fill the gap. This will change the number of currently enrolled nursing students (300,000) to the ideal number of enrolled students needed (400,000). The NLN projects the future need of full-time faculty members may be as high as 40,000. In the United States, there is currently reported to be about 20,000 full-time faculty members.

The National League for Nursing proposes that more attention should be given to the teaching component of the nursing role. It is important that all nurse educators know about teaching, learning, and evaluation. Academic nurse educators must have the skills and adequate knowledge needed to perform curriculum development, assessment of program outcomes, and to be an effective member of the academic community. More attention needs to be directed towards developing the science of nursing education. In order to develop well-prepared nursing educators, nurses should be prepared through a master's and/or doctoral education program, post-master's certificate program, and continue their professional development through various continuing education opportunities. Well-prepared nurse educators may become that way through mentoring by more experienced faculty, and through professional certification. Schools that offer such nurse educator post-degree programs should be commended, supported, and rewarded.

Encouraging professional development

The National League for Nursing has proposed several recommendations which will help to encourage nursing faculty to develop professionally. These recommendations include the following:
- Nursing schools should support life-long learning activities, which help educators maintain and expand their expertise in teaching and education, along with the clinical competence and scholarly skills.
- Schools should recognize and reward expert educators.
- Schools should support educators financially, strive to reduce workload, and provide support in developing their teaching, advisement, and program development skills.

- Schools of nursing should reward educators for designing innovative curricula, or developing creative ways to facilitate learning in the nursing student.

Attracting nurses to nursing education field

According to the NLN Board of Governors, several recommendations were approved as necessary in May 2002 to increase the number of nurse educators in the future. First of all, nurses should take advantage of the many opportunities which are available to prepare them as nurse educators. Mentoring by senior faculty should be provided to nurses who are new to education. Faculty should strive to promote careers in nursing education by identifying those students who demonstrate talent and by recruiting experienced clinicians who have demonstrated talent in education. Master's programs should offer a track that prepares beginning nurse educators for various roles, or that help clinician's make the transition to educator. Doctoral programs should strive to offer an option to students who choose to specialize in nursing education, and thus conduct research which is related to this specialized field.

Important terms

Science of nursing education: The science of education, or pedagogy, is the art or science of being a teacher/instructor/educator. The term *science of nursing education* refers to the strategies or style of instruction used to educate future nurses. It is the systematic process of instructing, learning, and employing the operations involved with accomplishing the task of educating nurses. This particular science focuses on graduate competencies of a nurse, expected nursing program outcomes, utilizing clinical teaching models, and providing effective nursing student advisement. It also involves the process of recruiting and retaining students for the nursing program, so they may become future nurse leaders and adequately prepared nursing clinicians.

Socialization to the role of nursing educator: This is the process in which a new nurse educator becomes familiar with the details and requirements of his or her new role as an educator. It usually will involve understanding a historical perspective of the role and the legal parameters inherent in the role. This socialization will occur through formal education, mentoring, and on-the-job experience.

Structured preparation for the faculty role: The formal systematic preparation of a future educator. Future educators must become familiar and adopt the core knowledge and skills required for their role. The future educator must have the ability to facilitate learning, advance the nursing student's development and professional socialization to nursing, design appropriate learning experiences, and evaluate outcomes. Future educators must also have the knowledge to skillfully develop nursing curriculum, assess program outcomes, and be an effective member of the academic community.

Pedagogical research: The systematic investigation into the teaching/learning process. It involves research and inquiry on how students learn, teaching strategies that are effective, proven evaluation methods, development and implementation of the curriculum, and environments which promote behavior change and thus learning in the student.

Scholarship, Service, and Leadership

Motivation to participate in professional development

Motivation is a term used to describe methods that can instigate behavior, direct and give purpose to behavior, encourage behavior to continue, and eventually will lead to choosing a particular behavior. The educator must perceive there is an advantage to attending the program. He or she must find the information valuable in order to change behavior. The educator's needs should be identified. The offered professional development activities should also serve the needs of the organization. Adults have a need for control over their learning choices. For faculty to participate, they must be able to make their own choices about their development opportunities. Many professional development opportunities offered to faculty propose changes to the way they have taught their students for many years. If they do not believe that the new method will enhance their professional life, or if it is perceived there is little support or reward for changing, they will not see the need to attend or learn the new method.

Adult learning

In order for adult learning to occur, certain principles should be followed to increase the nurse educator's effectiveness. The educator should create a climate of respect. In order to accomplish this, the student's characteristics, learning styles, academic and educational training, and their unique professional perspective should be considered. They should be encouraged to actively participate in the learning process. The educator should build on the adult student's experience. It is important to engage the students and have them share their experiences. A spirit of collaborative inquiry should be promoted by the educator. This is accomplished by utilizing small groups in the classroom and involving the students in assessing the needs of the group. The participants will need to learn for action. Educators can provide an atmosphere of support in which the student can try out the new behavior. Finally, by perceiving that they are able to change their environment and bring about a positive effect by their new behavior, the students will be empowered.

Needs assessment for new programs

A needs assessment should always be performed for the development of a new program. A needs assessment should also be done if there has been a change in the demographics of the population or the particular learning needs of health agency staff. It will also need to be revised if there is a change in the health status of the general population, or there is an anticipated health need in the community due to emerging issues or threats. Program revision will also need to be made in response to feedback from participants of previous programs. It is important for the nurse educator to assess external frame factors, which are factors which influence program development that come from outside the institution or clinic setting. Internal frame factors will also need to be assessed. These are the factors which affect the program from inside the clinic, agency, or home/work setting.

Community needs assessment
The nurse educator should describe the community with regard to its size, services, major industries, local government, and institutions of learning and religion. The demographics of the population should be evaluated. The community's employment environment—including income levels, percent of population with health insurance, education, and literacy levels, as well as languages spoken—should be assessed. The characteristics of the general family and household should also be identified. The community's health-promoting or health-damaging aspects of its environment will need to be identified, and the health and wellness measures of the general population should be calculated. Health-supporting institutions in the community should also be determined.

Guidelines for internal frame factors
The nurse educator will need to assess whether the mission, philosophy, and goals of the institution address staff development and health education needs. Is there congruency between the mission, philosophy, and goals of the program with that of the institution? The educator may assess the learning needs of the staff and/or patients using multiple information sources. The educator will need to determine the learning needs of the staff or clients to be served. The educator will also need to determine the characteristics of the staff or clients, in order to develop an appropriate program. Additionally, the institutional economics and resources for staff development and health education programs will need to be assessed. The educator will need to confirm that there are adequate resources for providing the programs.

Accreditation

Process
The accreditation process normally involves five elements. These elements usually include institutional self-study, peer review, site visit, and action by the accrediting association, and finally, the monitoring of the program. Self-study is the process of the institution evaluating itself, based on the provided standards of the accrediting association. Peer review will usually include stakeholders in the organization. It may be accomplished by faculty, key partners of the institution, administrators of the institution, and the public. The accrediting agency will perform site visits to clarify the self-study or self-analysis results, and provide any additional information necessary for evaluating the institution. All of the above information is provided to the accrediting agency, and a review by the agency is performed to determine whether accreditation is achieved. Programs are normally reviewed every 5-10

years with monitoring by the review of annual reports submitted to the accrediting agency by the institution.

Agencies and programs
The National League for Nursing Accreditation Agency accredits vocational, diploma, associate degree, baccalaureate and higher degree nursing programs. The National League for Nursing was the original accreditation agency, and was first established in 1952. The NLNAC established itself in 1998 as an outgrowth of that original agency. The Commission on Collegiate Nursing Education accredits baccalaureate and higher degree nursing programs. The Council on Accreditation of Nurse Anesthesia Educational Programs accredits nurse anesthesia educational programs at the certificate, masters and doctoral degree levels. The Division of Accreditation of the American College of Nurse Midwives accredits precertification, basic certificate, and master's degree nurse-midwifery educational programs. The Council on Accreditation for the National Association of Nurse Practitioners in Women's health accredits women's health nurse practitioner programs.

Doctoral degrees

There are four different kinds of doctoral degrees specifically awarded in nursing. The four degree types are the Doctor of Philosophy (PhD), the Education Doctorate (EdD), the Doctorate of Nursing Science (DNSc), and the Nursing Doctorate (ND). The PhD of nursing is considered a research-based degree, with the goal of advancing nursing practice research. The ND and the DNSc are considered professional degrees which specialize in clinical applications research. The EdD focuses mainly on the education of nurses, with research focused on issues related to nursing education. Currently, it is reported that only 0.6% of the registered nurse population have a doctorate degree.

Culturally diverse students

It is important for the culturally sensitive nurse educator to be aware of their own values, norms, and beliefs in regards to cultural diversity. The educator should understand how these perspectives will influence their view of life, family, and relationships. The professional educator should practice a respectful attitude to all cultures and the differences they will encompass. She or he should value the strengths and differences, rather than be critical of the differences. The educator should develop and promote continuing education about a predominant culture in their specific community or institution. The educator should utilize professionals from other cultures in order to learn more about the cultures. When change is being promoted, it is important to consider and understand how it will affect the culturally diverse student.

Organizational effectiveness

Organizational effectiveness is the concept of how effective an organization is in achieving their desired outcomes. It is an abstract concept which is difficult to measure. To assess or evaluate organization effectiveness in nursing education, the professional educator will need to obtain numerous proxy measures. These measures may include the number of students served by the institution and their demographics, the number of student graduates of nursing, and the number of graduates who pass the nursing boards. Current accreditation criteria emphasize program outcome evaluation. A particular outcome which might be required by the accrediting body might include the graduates to demonstrate the ability to communicate effectively, whereas the faculty of the organization may identify the satisfaction of students, graduates, employers, and patients as a valuable program outcome measure.

Master plan

A master plan is an outline of the standards and criteria required to evaluate a program's effectiveness. It will identify what criteria and standards will be analyzed and evaluated during and at the completion of the program. This allows the faculty to gather data on an ongoing basis, and thus determine if the program is on track to meet the expected outcomes or whether there may be a need to revise and improve the program on an ongoing basis. The master plan outlines the area to be evaluated, what the sources of data will be, the tools, instruments and any other methods which will be used for data collecting, the assessment time frame, who specifically will be responsible for each activity associated with the plan of evaluation, the specific criteria used to analyze if outcomes are being met, how to report results and how decisions will be made according to these results, and what the action plan will be to develop, maintain, and revise the program.

Community leadership

There are many roles nurse educators can take to provide leadership in the community where they live and teach. Nursing school faculty are obvious leaders, as their expertise may be sought by the surrounding health care community. Nurse educators may also serve as clinicians, researchers, administrators, and authors, as well as consultants, to provide such leadership. The Sigma Theta Tau International Honor Society of Nursing is an excellent resource to tap into in order to develop leadership skills and opportunities for leadership in the community. This society offers admission based on academic achievements by the nurse. Sigma Theta Tau International sponsors an International Leadership Academy. This academy offers nurse and honor society chapter leaders an opportunity to enhance their leadership skills. Members of Sigma Theta Tau International are a part of the second-largest nursing organization in the world, with approximately 125,000 active members. It exists to improve the health of people and increase the scientific base of nursing research.

Leadership in nursing programs

The American Association of Colleges of Nursing is an association which promotes advancing higher education in nursing. The AACN sponsors an executive leadership fellowship. This fellowship is designed to assist aspiring and new administrators of nursing education. It provides a program which develops skills in assessment and evaluation. It provides a wonderful opportunity for strategic networking within the nurse leadership community. It is a yearlong program which examines case studies related to successful leadership and opportunities to establish strong mentor and peer networks. GANES is a professional organization whose membership entails national associations of nursing deans and schools of nursing. It offers information, support, and advice to health care policymakers and nurse educators across the world.

Types of faculty scholarship

Ernest Boyer identified four interrelated types of faculty scholarship in his book, *Scholarship Reconsidered: Priorities of the Professoriate.* The four types are discovery or disciplinary research; application, or responsibly applying knowledge to societal needs and practice; integration, or interdisciplinary collaboration; and teaching, or the systematic approach to student learning through discovering what and how students learn. The six stages of scholarship include clear goals, adequate preparation, appropriate methods, significant results, effective presentation, and reflective technique. A scholar must state the purposes for the study clearly in order to establish clear goals. He or she should be prepared with knowledge gathered extensively with regard to the study. Are appropriate methods used which will help the scholar reach the desired goals? Are the results significant to the selected field of study? Are the results presented with clarity and integrity? The scholar should critically evaluate his or her own work.

Change

Positive approach for implementation

In order to direct successful change within an organization, it is important for the educator to understand the process necessary to implement change. It is important to develop stakeholders within the organization. Stakeholders are people who have been given the opportunity to provide input, and have bought into the idea of change. Remember that resistance is often a sign that change is beginning to occur. Educators need to address any lack of understanding in order to address this resistance. Remember that culture may be a basis for change to be rejected. You may need to change the change, or change the culture. You will need to develop trust among the recipients of change. Make sure that the perceived level of commitment to the change by the leadership of the organization is well communicated. Remember that discomfort in the way that things have always been done will often be a strong driving force of change. There must be a certain reward identified by people for making the change.

Empirical-rational change strategy

When utilizing this change strategy, it is assumed that people are rational beings and they will follow their own self-interest. To enact successful change, the identified change must be communicated well and incentives need to be offered. If incentives are only modest, this change may be difficult to achieve. If the leader of change can convince those involved of the need for change, there is a greater likelihood of success. It is important to develop stakeholders who are viewed with respect or power within the organization. These stakeholders can be instrumental in selling, promoting, and convincing others of the needed change.

Normative-reeducative change strategy

When utilizing this change strategy, it is assumed that people are social beings and they will adhere to cultural norms and values. It is important for the educator to develop commitments to new values and norms by redefining and reinterpreting the old ones. It is also important for the educator to cultivate charisma and dynamic leadership to bring about this type of change. To effect change, the educator must focus on the organization's culture. Culture change often occurs slowly. It is important to enlist and involve the informal leaders of the organization in order to incorporate the normative-reeducative actions for change.

Power-coercive change strategy

When utilizing this change strategy, it is assumed that people are basically compliant and will generally do what they are told or made to do. Change may be brought about by this method by exercising authority and establishing sanctions. With this type of change management, those that are affected by the change are given few options. The main reasons for adopting this approach are a lack of time and the potential of a serious threat. People must be convinced that the old way of doing things will cause collapse in the organization, and thus this new change must take effect immediately.

Environmental-adaptive change strategy

When utilizing this change strategy, it is assumed that people oppose loss and disruption, but that they will adapt readily to new circumstances. This change strategy seeks to put the burden of the change onto the people of an organization, as opposed to the management of the organization. It attempts to avoid the difficulties of trying to change the people or culture of an organization. This strategy attempts to create a new organization, rather than try to change the old one. This type of strategy works best when there is a need for radical, transformative change.

Selecting change strategy

The nurse educator will need to consider the degree of change that is needed within an organization. If a radical change is needed, then the environmental-adaptive strategy should be chosen, but should not be used if a less radical change is needed. If strong resistance is expected, then a possible coupling of power-coercive and environmental-adaptive change may be needed. If weak resistance is expected, then a combination of rational-empirical and normative-reeducative strategies may be needed. Population will determine strategy, in that large or diverse populations may need a mix of all four strategies. Stakes will also determine choice, in that high stakes may require a mix of all four strategies. Moderate or low stakes should not utilize the power-coercive strategy. Short time frames need a power-coercive strategy. Longer time frames may mix rational-empirical, normative-reeducative, and environmental-adaptive. If there is adequate expertise, then a mix of strategies may be utilized but if inadequate, the educator may need to rely on power-coercive.

Supporting change

A professional nurse educator may be instrumental in supporting changes within her or his organization and in this way, may bring about needed changes and be an agent for proactive change. When change is presented as needed by the organization, the nurse educator leader should become fully educated about the change and how it should be brought about. The educator can ask questions and clarify information with regard to the promoted change. Once the educator is knowledgeable about the change and understands its need, then he or she can take on stakeholder status. The educator has then bought into the need for change, and can be an advocate for it by informing others within the organization and addressing issues which arise during the process of change. The educator can immediately adopt the changes and put them into practice. In this way, the educator is becoming a role model for the change and demonstrating its feasibility.

Modeling positive attitude

As a leader of students and professional peers, the nurse educator should demonstrate a positive attitude towards change. The nurse educator must understand and accept that change is constant. Priorities, resources, and people are in a constant flux. Nurse educator leaders must model resilience, flexibility, and the ability to adapt as change occurs. Others will watch the nurse educator's reaction to shifting priorities, changing policies, diminishing resources, and changing demands on precious time. It is important to maintain open communication during the process of change. Communication lines must be open in order to let people know exactly what is happening and why. Open communication will allow for questions and concerns to be shared by others, so that they will be well-informed as to the what, why, and how of the pending change. As a leader, ask the question to yourself and others: "How can we get better at adapting to change?"

Legal actions/decisions and practice standards applied to ethical principles

The ethical principle of autonomy could be linked with the Cardozo decision regarding informed content, institutional review boards, the Patient Self-Determination Act, the Patient's Bill of Rights, and the Joint Commission standards. The ethical principle of veracity, or truth telling, may be linked with the Tuma decision, the Patient's Bill of Rights, Joint Commission standards and the Cardozo decision. The ethical principle of confidentiality may be linked with privileged information standards, the Patient's Bill of Rights, HIPAA, and Joint Commission standards.

The ethical principle of nonmalfeasance could be linked with malpractice/negligence rights and duties, nurse practice acts, the Patient's Bill of Rights, *Darling v. Charleston Memorial Hospital*, state health codes, and Joint Commission standards. The ethical principle of beneficence could be linked with the Patient's Bill of Rights, state health codes, job descriptions, standards of practice, policy and procedure manuals, and Joint Commission standards. Justice may be linked with the Patient's Bill of Rights, antidiscrimination/affirmative action laws, the Americans with Disabilities Act, and Joint Commission standards. These laws and professional standards help to ensure that every person's fundamental rights are being acknowledged and honored.

FERPA

FERPA is the Family Educational Rights and Privacy Act of 1974. It is a federal law which gives students certain rights in regards to their educational records. Student test-takers have the right to expect that certain information about them will be kept confidential. It is the responsibility of the educator to assure that the student's privacy is maintained with regard to testing scores and education records. The educator should be aware that students are allowed to review their academic records, which are maintained by the school. The student has the right to request that the school correct records which they believe are inaccurate or just misleading. The educator should be aware that the school must have written permission from the student to release any information from the student's record. FERPA limits access to records to those who have rights to the information to meet the student's educational requirements.

Codes of ethical conduct

Several codes have been developed by professional associations to protect the student when undergoing testing and/or various assessments. Some of these codes include: the Code of Fair Testing Practices in Education, the Code of Professional Responsibilities in Educational Measurement, and the 9 Principles of Good Practice for Assessing Student Learning from the American Association for Higher Education, and the Standards for Educational and Psychological Testing. The nurse educator should be aware of the common elements of these codes and standards. Teachers are responsible for the test quality and the selection of appropriate tests for their student population. Fair test administration procedures should be followed to protect the safety, health, and welfare of all students. Teachers are responsible for the accurate scoring of these tests, and feedback and results of testing should be provided in a timely manner.

ADA

The ADA, otherwise known as the Americans with Disabilities Act of 1990, was developed to protect disabled Americans in many different ways. With regard to evaluation of students with disabilities, the nursing educator must be aware of the importance of honoring this act. The law prohibits discrimination against qualified individuals with disabilities. Qualified individuals with disabilities may meet the requirements to be admitted to a nursing program. It will be up to the nursing program to accommodate this individual with regard to any physical needs or aids. The nursing program will need to provide reasonable accommodations, and remove any barriers to learning. Such reasonable accommodations may include oral testing, extended time for exams, test readers, sign language interpreters, large print or type for tests, and possibly a private testing area.

Scholarship of Teaching

Community development approach to scholarship

Research studies have been done which suggest the advantages of creating a community development approach to scholarship among nursing educators. Rather than creating a competitive environment among faculty peers or within the educator with regard to balancing research with teaching; a collaborative approach is sought. In this way, the individual scholarly accomplishments are not the desired goal, but instead a collaborative effort by scholars supporting each other and working together to achieve scholarship results. To achieve the goal of collaborative research, it is important to develop a spirit of sharing and mutual goal attainment. It must be acknowledged that different scholars bring different areas of expertise to the table. It is important to value each nurse educator's interests, knowledge, and experiences. Avenues for promoting sharing of ideas should be utilized, such as face-to-face meetings, teleconferences, and general space for conversations.

Building scholarship capacity

The researchers Lansang and Dennis promote four approaches to building research capacity among scholars. First, it is important to prepare scholars academically to undertake research. This can be accomplished through training programs, which train scholars in specific research skills, such as grant writing. Mentorships are another approach to building scholarship. Mentorships among colleagues working one-on-one to provide training and support to one another are important to increase research capacity. The creation of research excellence centers will provide leadership in specialized fields of study. Teams working together to create a scholarly project provides another approach. These teams should partner to provide information from different professional educators, with regard to their expertise and experiences.

Collaboration to build scholarship community of educators

There are many advantages for nursing educators who work together with colleagues to create scholarship in their community. When faculty members work together towards a common goal of scholarship, much can be accomplished, and many advantages are gained by this partnership. It is important to obtain differing viewpoints and ideas; brainstorming about a common issue is much more productive among one's scholarly peers, as opposed to working individually. One wonderful advantage is a sense of camaraderie and collegiality. Just having the opportunity to discuss an issue of scholarship with colleagues is an advantage. It prevents a feeling of isolation in performing one's scholarly work. It also offers an opportunity to connect and network among professional colleagues.

Scholarship of teaching

Scholarship of teaching, scholarship, and scholarly method are similar terms. Essentially, it is the body of principles and practices used by scholars (educators) to make their claims about their world as trustworthy and valid. Scholarship publications provide the instrument to make these claims public to the scholarship world or academic population. It is the body of knowledge accrued by research in a particular field (in this case, teaching and specifically, in teaching of nurses). Works of scholarship are often published in professional journals. As an academic nurse educator, it is important to develop an area of expertise in this role. This will mean not only teaching nursing students, but performing research in relation to the best way to disseminate this information and create highly skilled, knowledgeable nurses.

Evidence-based resources

Evidence-based resources are resources which are based on scientifically proven evidence. These resources are based on reports from multiple research studies, individual randomized clinical trials, and non-experimental research. By utilizing evidence-based resources, the researcher or student will avoid subjective concerns of nonresearch-based evidence. Evidence-based resources are the type of evidence which is generally considered stronger evidence. It is usually research brought about by carefully designed and implemented research. Such research reports will include an introduction or problem, methods used to gather data about this particular problem, the results of the data gathering, and finally, the conclusions, interpretations or discussion of the results.

Scholarly paper

A scholarly paper is an academic work which is usually published in a specialized academic journal. It should contain either original research results, or reviews of other research results. It may also be referred to as an article. If a paper is to be considered for publication, it must undergo a peer review by academics in the same field as the topic of the paper. In this way, the paper is checked as to its suitability for publication. Unfortunately, it is often a time-intensive process to become published. The paper must undergo reviews, edits, and re-submissions before it is either accepted or rejected for publication. Then, once it is accepted, it may not appear in the journal of submission for up to a year, due to the extensive number of articles awaiting publication in that particular journal. It is important for the author of the article to cite sources used, so that credit to other authors whose work they have utilized for their article can be given.

Function Effectively in Community

Community college vs. four-year college or university setting

Community colleges are considered to be primarily teaching institutions. The main mission of the community college is to educate the local population, and thus provide skilled workers for the surrounding workforce. The faculty duties of a community college's instructors are usually two-fold, involving mostly teaching and service. The faculty duties of instructors at a four year institution of learning are usually three-fold. The nurse educator working in this environment will be expected to not only teach and provide service, but also to develop scholarship (research and publication). The four year college nursing instructor will be expected to incorporate research into their classes. In community colleges, service by the educator will be expected to be provided to the surrounding community. In the four year college or university, the expectations of service are to the institution itself.

College or university vs. research-intensive university

The teaching load is often heavier in a college or university which is primarily a teaching institution. The teaching load may vary on whether the nursing instructor is educating the undergraduate or graduate nurse. In some institutions, the same nursing faculty may be responsible for teaching some undergraduate and graduate nursing courses. Often, graduate nursing faculty members will have a lighter teaching load, due to the fact their research requirements are higher. The graduate nursing instructor may need to also be available to the graduate nursing students to mentor through the thesis and dissertation process. In some states or institutions,

- 73 -

union regulations may require certain terms with regard to teaching load. Whether required to be a member of the union or not, instructors will still be affected by the negotiated terms.

Committees

A committee is a small deliberative assembly which may serve different functions in order to accomplish a task, solve an assigned problem, or achieve a particular goal as a group. Some of the functions served include research and recommendations, governance, project management, and coordination of a larger group. A nurse educator may volunteer to serve, or be appointed to a committee. These committees may be departmental or university-wide (teaching institution-wide). The nurse educator, when volunteering, may need to decide what committees to choose to serve. It is important to choose committees in which the educators' strengths will be an asset and an effective contribution will be provided. Institutions and their subsequent departments usually expect their professional educators to participate in committee work. This is one aspect of the professional nurse educator's responsibilities as an academic member.

Information Age

In modern times, often known as the Information Age, access to extensive amounts of information is readily available to the student. In the past, the educator was often sought as the main source of information. Today, students can simply perform an Internet search to obtain the information they might be seeking. Thus, the instructor is no longer the sole source responsible for imparting knowledge to the student. The educator's role has changed so that he or she serves a role as a facilitator of knowledge, as opposed to the imparter of knowledge. For this reason, educators must develop a collaborative atmosphere between the teacher and the student. Memorization is becoming a less important form of learning; instead, educators seek to help their students learn how to refine a problem, discover the information they need to solve it, and to critically evaluate the discovered information.

ADA of 1990

The ADA has brought about many wonderful changes to the quality of life and the health future of individuals with disabilities. Unfortunately, there are an increasing number of disabled people in the population. Their disabilities may have been caused by a birth defect, an injury, or a disease which may be permanent in nature. This population will need assistance from the nurse educator in transitioning from being a recipient of care to performing their own self-care, and becoming responsible for their own wellness to maintain their optimum level of functioning. The disabled population may have overt physical disabilities, or they may have a cognitive or mental impairment that may be difficult to detect. The disabled student often presents complex needs. The nurse educator will play an integral role as part of an interdisciplinary team effort to assist these individuals. The nurse educator must be aware of the barrier to learning that exists for their clients, and should be knowledgeable about available interventions and technologies to overcome these barriers.

Learning disabilities

There are an ever-increasing number of learning disabilities, which include such identified learning hindrances as attention deficit disorders, memory deficits, integrative processing disorders, visual and auditory perceptual disabilities, minimal brain dysfunction, and developmental language problems. In the past, learning disabilities were expected to be outgrown, but it is being discovered that most individuals do not outgrow their learning disabilities. It is the responsibility of the nurse educator to become well-versed in understanding these various types of disabilities and to become familiar with assistive technologies and teaching strategies that will facilitate learning in this population.

ADHD
ADHD is a disability which may include one or more of these characteristics: hyperactivity, lack of attention or inattention, and impulsivity. Boys often outnumber girls by three to one with the incidence of this disorder. About 50% of these diagnosed individuals will grow out of this disorder, but sometimes a diagnosis of ADDRET is maintained. ADDRET is Attention Deficit Disorder Residual Type, an affliction where the affected individuals are no longer hyperactive, but may continue to experience problems of a different but related nature. Those with this disability tend to be disorganized, exhibit sloppy handwriting, and be poor time managers. The nurse educator may assist these individuals by providing a quiet atmosphere to learn new information, breaking up directions into small steps, rewarding achievement, attempting to ignore inappropriate behavior, and eliminating distractions as much as possible.

Practice Test

Practice Questions

1. When preparing a lesson regarding culturally sensitive care, the nurse educator should begin with which of the following?
    a. Becoming familiar with the learners' cultures
    b. Examining and considering personal culture
    c. Identifying cultural adaptations made by learners
    d. Noting specific cultural differences between the nurse educator and the learners

2. The nurse educator recognizes that the learners in the associate-degree nursing program have more limited job opportunities than those with BSNs. Which of the following is the best advice to give learners in the program?
    a. Transfer to a BSN program in lieu of the AS degree program.
    b. Plan to look for employment only in the training hospitals and facilities.
    c. Take the AS program only if you plan to live and work in the state.
    d. Consider taking an RN-to-BSN bridge program after graduation.

3. The clinical nurse educator notes that one learner in a first clinical rotation has a high threat perception and is too frightened to adequately provide care to clients. Which of the following is the best initial intervention?
    a. Assign the learner to work with a preceptor.
    b. Accompany the learner throughout the clinical experience.
    c. Ask the learner to write a reflective journal about fear.
    d. Remove the learner from the clinical rotation for the present.

4. The nurse educator is in a leadership position and finds that one member of the staff is performing below expectations. What is the first action that the nurse educator should take when meeting with the staff member?
    a. Explain how the person's behavior is affecting staff performance.
    b. Describe the behavior that requires change.
    c. Outline the steps that the staff member needs to take.
    d. Advise the person of the consequences for failure to make changes.

5. Because of a shortage of qualified nurse educators, the board has advised the school of nursing to develop computer-based training (CBT) to replace some traditional classes. Which of the following courses best lends itself to development as computer-based training?
    a. Information and technology literacy
    b. Nursing ethics
    c. Theories of teaching and learning
    d. Foundations of nursing

6. An experienced nurse educator meets with a novice nurse educator who is going to teach a course that the experienced nurse educator has taught a number of times. The novice nurse educator expresses concern about being behind schedule in developing the course outline, course content, and examinations. Which of the following is the best response by the experienced nurse educator?
    a. Suggest the novice nurse utilize the experienced nurse's materials.
    b. Empathize about how difficult it is to prepare for courses.
    c. Suggest that the novice nurse discuss the problem with the program director.
    d. Ask the novice nurse if the experienced nurse can assist in some way.

7. When plotting learner scores on a Bell curve, what percentage of learner scores does the nurse educator expect will fall within one standard deviation of the mean?
    a. 33%
    b. 68%
    c. 95%
    d. 99%

8. A nurse educator has completed a grant-writing workshop and wants to apply for a large federal grant to increase the integration of technology into nursing education and clinical practice. What is the first item the nurse educator should do before beginning the application process?
    a. Ask an experienced grant writer for advice.
    b. Read carefully through the grant application.
    c. Read through a number of successful grant applications.
    d. Begin to gather necessary evidence and materials.

9. According to the National League for Nursing's *Excellence in Nursing Education Model©*, what comprises a "well-prepared faculty"?
    a. A faculty with expertise in different areas
    b. A faculty comprised of researchers
    c. A faculty with degrees in nursing education
    d. A faculty comprised of expert clinicians

10. According to the Kolb Learning Style Inventory, which type of learning experience does the learner with an assimilative style likely prefer?
    a. Concrete experiences and active experimentation
    b. Concrete experiences and reflective observation
    c. Abstract conceptualization and active administration
    d. Abstract conceptualization and reflective observation

11. Which of the following shows the most consistent commitment to lifelong learning?
    a. The nurse educator plans to obtain a doctorate degree at some time in the future.
    b. The nurse educator completes required continuing education courses.
    c. The nurse educator reads professional journals and is taking an Internet course.
    d. The nurse educator attends a nursing conference annually.

12. Which of the following is the best activity to promote one's socialization in the role of nurse educator?
    a. Participate in meetings, committees, and other professional activities.
    b. Invite fellow staff members to one's home for a party or dinner.
    c. Arrange for after-hours activities, such as bowling, with other staff.
    d. Serve as a mentor to a novice nurse educator.

13. During the obstetrics clinical rotation, a number of clients who were assigned male nursing learners objected to receiving care from men, preventing the male nursing learners from obtaining necessary experience. Which of the following is the best approach for the nurse educator in solving this problem?
    a. Increase simulation training for male nursing learners
    b. Tell clients that they do not have a choice about the nurse's gender
    c. Ask clients in advance if they feel comfortable with a male nurse
    d. Allow the male nurses more time to complete the rotation

14. The nurse educator is preparing a content item worksheet for the first four weeks of the course, which meets four hours weekly. Based on this worksheet, the nurse educator will determine how many test questions should cover each unit on the midterm exam, which will have a total of 50 questions:

	Unit 1	Unit 2
Lecture hours	10	6
% of lecture hours	60%	40%
Number of exam items	?	?

Based on this worksheet, how many test exam items should the nurse educator write to cover the material in unit 2?
   a. 6
   b. 10
   c. 20
   d. 40

15. When discussing diversity with a group of learners, the nurse educator asks the learners to consider whether people's beliefs and practices could only be accurately judged from within the context of their own cultures. Which of the following terms does this idea represent?
   a. Ethnocentrism
   b. Cultural relativism
   c. Cultural competence
   d. Cultural awareness

16. The nurse educator at a community college is interested in forming an articulation agreement with a nearby university so that the learners in the RN program can receive a BSN, a process that is allowed in the state. Which of the following should the nurse educator do first?
   a. Take the proposal to the director of the school of nursing.
   b. Take the proposal to the college president.
   c. Take the proposal to the board of trustees.
   d. Take the proposal to the appropriate dean.

17. In story-based learning, *letting learn* refers to which of the following?
   a. Providing learners adequate time and multiple opportunities to master material.
   b. Allowing learners to share stories that are inspiring and providing lessons about caring from their own experience.
   c. Allowing learners to determine what information is needed and to acquire knowledge for purpose.
   d. Providing a detailed outline of content for students but allowing them to find resources to study independently.

18. The nurse educator has developed items for an assessment test that covers four chapters in the textbook. There are 100 items in five different types: essay, short answer, completion, multiple choice, and true/false. When organizing the test, how should the nurse educator group the test items?
   a. By content
   b. By chapter
   c. By difficulty
   d. By type

19. The nurse educator developed a trial mentoring program during the last semester of the senior year for graduating nurses to determine if learners who participated in the mentoring program had higher NCLEX scores than those who attended NCLEX preparation workshops in the learning lab. Learners were randomly assigned with half to one group and half to the other.

Using the PSCOT (population, strategy, comparison, outcome, time) method of questioning evidence-based teaching, how would the nurse educator outline this question?

	a.	b.	c.	d.
P	Graduating nurses	Graduating nurses	Graduating nurses	Graduating nurses
S	Mentoring	Workshops	Intervention A	50%
C	NCLEX Workshops	Mentoring	Intervention B	50%
O	NCLEX score	NCLEX score	NCLEX score	NCLEX score
T	Last semester	Last semester	Last semester	Last semester

20. According to Herzberg's (1968) theory of motivation, what is the primary factor leading to satisfaction with one's job?
   a. Increased compensation
   b. Job security
   c. Advancement opportunities
   d. Congenial environment

21. Which type of empowerment is derived from sharing new techniques and healthcare news from research and Internet searches with peers?
   a. Informational
   b. Rewarding
   c. Connecting
   d. Referent

22. Which of the following instructional methods is the best approach to teaching a psychomotor skill?

 a. Discuss the underlying principles of the process while teaching the learners the steps to carry out the skill.

 b. Ask the learners to focus on their feelings about the process while carrying out the steps to the process.

 c. Ask the learners how they would best like to approach learning a psychomotor skill.

 d. Focus only on the steps to carrying out the psychomotor skill and discuss principles and feelings at another time.

23. When researching evidence-based teaching strategies, which of the following databases would be most useful?

 a. Best Health

 b. CINAHL

 c. The Cochrane Library

 d. Health Systems Evidence

24. During a clinical experience, a learner who concludes that a client has had poor self-management of diabetes because of decreasing vision rather than willful lack of compliance is exhibiting which level of cognitive behavior?

 a. Analysis

 b. Evaluation

 c. Application

 d. Synthesis

25. Which of the following is the primary purpose of a curriculum philosophy statement?

 a. Outline specific goals and objectives.

 b. Describe the curriculum in the program.

 c. Explain the purpose of the education program.

 d. Guide curriculum development.

26. According to the Synergy Model when applied to education, which learner characteristic refers to the learner's adaptability to differences in teaching styles and strategies and different styles of learning?

 a. Readiness

 b. Vulnerability

 c. Resilience

 d. Predictability

27. A nurse educator is serving as the clinical instructor for a group of learners in the medical-surgical department. What is the primary role of the clinical instructor?
   a. Supervising
   b. Guiding and facilitating learning
   c. Teaching
   d. Preventing medical or treatment errors

28. According to Boyer, "scholarship of discovery" refers to which of the following?
   a. Completing original research
   b. Connecting theory to practice
   c. Interpreting and synthesizing knowledge
   d. Providing evidence of effective teaching

29. When developing competency statements as part of curricular design, the nurse educator must consider three elements: the right learner, the right behavior, and which of the following?
   a. Right tools
   b. Right resources
   c. Right time frame
   d. Right context

30. When evaluating program effectiveness in terms of organization of curriculum, the principle of *vertical organization* refers to which of the following?
   a. Sequencing of courses and levels of complexity
   b. Organizing a hierarchy (board to faculty)
   c. Identifying the extent to which the elements of the program fit together
   d. Identifying needed skills at each level of the curriculum

31. Which of the following is the purpose of using MeSH code?
   a. To send messages via the Internet
   b. To prevent hacking of Internet accounts
   c. To facilitate searching in PubMed and other databases
   d. To organize files on a computer into different domains

32. According to Keller's (1987) ARCS model for creating a motivating learning environment, which of the following refers to learning requirements, difficulty level, learner expectations, and sense of accomplishment?
   a. Attention
   b. Relevance
   c. Confidence
   d. Satisfaction

33. A nurse educator assesses learners at the beginning of each class for learning styles and learning needs. Which of the National League for Nursing's Nurse Educator Competencies does this support?
    a. Facilitate learning
    b. Facilitate learner development and socialization
    c. Use assessment and evaluation strategies
    d. Pursue continuous quality improvement

34. After conducting surveys as part of outreach to an underrepresented ethnic minority, the nurse educator finds that, despite the desire of many to enroll in nursing school, enrollment is low because the majority of learners work in low-paying jobs during the daytime when classes are in session and cannot afford to quit work to attend school fulltime. Which is the best solution for the school of nursing?
    a. Target a different group of potential learners
    b. Increase financial aid to the underrepresented group
    c. Offer classes in the evening and/or online and part-time admission
    d. Increase advertisement and outreach to the underrepresented group

35. Algorithms are most useful when teaching which type of course content?
    a. Skills
    b. Concepts
    c. Issues
    d. Theories

36. A nurse educator who has a good sense of humor, cares about learners, and serves as a mentor is exhibiting which type of competency?
    a. Scholarship
    b. Professional practice
    c. Service and faculty governance
    d. Relationships with learners/colleagues

37. The nurse educator plans to use debate as a teaching strategy to help learners develop analytical skills. Which of the following would be the most effective topic for debate?
    a. Traditional vs. microsurgical techniques.
    b. Assisted suicide for the terminally ill.
    c. Advantages of the Affordable Care Act.
    d. The use of simulation in the learning lab.

38. When reviewing a textbook, the nurse educator notes that the chapters about hypertension, obesity, and diabetes have only brief or no references to African Americans, who are at high risk for these health problems. Which type of bias does this represent?
    a. Stereotyping
    b. Imbalance/Selectivity
    c. Omission/Invisibility
    d. Isolation/Fragmentation

39. Which of the following characteristics is most representative of Millennials/Generation Y (born 1981 to 2003)?
    a. Flexible and able to multitask well but pessimistic.
    b. Self-centered and resistant to compromise but proactive.
    c. Rule-oriented, trustworthy, and practical.
    d. Rule followers, optimistic, socially involved, and team players.

40. When using the learner results of the Myers-Briggs Type Indicator to determine the ways in which the learner perceives and processes information, which of the following learning preferences might the nurse educator expect of a learner whose preference is for introversion rather than extroversion?
    a. Likes a quiet space without interruptions
    b. Likes group work
    c. Likes fast-paced learning
    d. Shares opinions readily without being asked

41. Which of the following is an example of a behavioral objective in the affective domain at the *characterization* level?
    a. During a group evaluation process following a group presentation, the learner will discuss feelings associated with the activity.
    b. Upon completion of the diabetic testing module, the learner will express confidence in the ability to carry out testing and interpret findings.
    c. Following a series of class sessions about ethics and confidentiality, the learner will show consistent interest in respecting client's rights and protecting confidentiality.
    d. After completing the module on calculating drip rates, the learner will be able to do calculations accurately.

42. Which three variables should the nurse educator consider when choosing instructional materials?
    a. Learner, media, and task.
    b. Time, costs, and equipment.
    c. Audience, literacy, and layout.
    d. Print, demonstration, and audiovisual.

43. The nurse educator has administered learning styles inventories to a class of 28 learners. The results show the following:

        Visual learners: 13
        Auditory learners: 6
        Kinesthetic learners: 3
        Mixed visual/auditory: 5

Based on these findings, which of the following approaches to teaching should the nurse educator focus on?

    a. Provide written materials, charts, diagrams, and videos that learners can read and observe.
    b. Provide written materials, graphs, charts, and videos; give explanations, answer questions, and provide materials for manipulation.
    c. Provide explanations and audiotapes and allow time for questions and answers.
    d. Provide materials for the learners to manipulate and provide minimal written or spoken information.

44. At a class level, which of the following is the best method to assess a learner's cognitive knowledge base at the beginning of a course of study, such as for topics in medical-surgical nursing?

    a. Ask the learner to do demonstrations.
    b. Administer a pretest to the learner.
    c. Conduct a learning styles inventory.
    d. Conduct a survey about the learner's previous studies.

45. The nurse educator had a difficult semester, encountering conflicts with a small group of learners who had been out of school for many years and disliked group projects. This conflict was reflected in their learner evaluations, which assessed the nurse educator as a poor communicator with deficient teaching skills. Which of the following is the best response when reviewing the evaluations with the director of the program?

    a. Point out that the negative evaluations were from a small group of unhappy learners.
    b. Note that the learners were resentful because they received low grades on group projects.
    c. Acknowledge the need to develop better strategies for teaching non-traditional learners.
    d. Ask the director about the best approach for dealing with difficult learners in the classroom.

46. The nurse educator has noted that one learner has exhibited repeated acts of annoying behavior, such as arriving late to class, failing to turn in assignments on time, and being rude to other learners. Which proactive measure is most important?
    a. Warn the learner regarding behavior
    b. Report the learner to administration
    c. Refer the learner for counseling
    d. Document observations

47. To which domain of learning is lecture and one-on-one instruction directed?
    a. Cognitive domain
    b. Affective domain
    c. Psychomotor domain
    d. Both cognitive and affective domain

48. The concept of *distributed practice* (Willingham, 2002) refers to which of the following?
    a. Doing clinical practice in a number of different places.
    b. Alternating clinical practice with classwork and individual study.
    c. Learning information over a number of successive time periods.
    d. Learning information all at once, such as during one cramming session.

49. According to Krathwohl et al.'s (1964) levels of affective behavior, which level is a learner exhibiting when the learner shows a willingness to focus on data and shows awareness of an idea?
    a. Characterization
    b. Valuing
    c. Responding
    d. Receiving

50. A learner who develops a more efficient method of using a piece of medical equipment during clinical experience is exhibiting psychomotor behavior at which level?
    a. Adaptation
    b. Origination
    c. Mechanism
    d. Perception

51. As part of the teaching plan, the nurse educator outlines the plan of teaching learners to administer heparin, including identifying sites, drawing up medication, administering the medication, and expressing concerns, using a human model for the demonstration. Which of the following methods of evaluation is most appropriate to evaluate the administration portion of the procedure?
    a. Return demonstration
    b. Post-test
    c. Question and answers
    d. Essay

52. A learner has negotiated a learning contract with the nurse educator for the service-learning component of the class; however, at the half-way point in the semester, the learner has completed only 20% of the activities while 50% should be completed. Which of the following is the best solution?
    a. Warn the learner that failure to complete the contract will result in a failing grade.
    b. Ask the learner to explain why he or she is not fulfilling the terms of the contract.
    c. Discuss with the learner the problems he or she is having completing the contract.
    d. Cancel the contract and make assignments to ensure the learner completes the activities.

53. A newly-hired novice educator believes that processes in place are inefficient and immediately suggests a number of changes. Which of the following should the nurse educator expect from other staff members?
    a. Anger
    b. Resistance
    c. Appreciation
    d. Compliance

54. Learners have a right to both procedural and substantive due process when they face disciplinary action or academic concerns. Which of the following is related to *substantive* due process?
    a. The right to be heard.
    b. The right to notification of concerns.
    c. The right to a hearing.
    d. The right to nondiscriminatory decisions.

55. The nursing school has been successful in attracting ethnic minorities to its program, but many of the learners speak English as a second language and have such strong accents that other healthcare providers and clients have difficulty understanding them at times. Which of the following is the best solution?
    a. Require a spoken test of English as a prerequisite for admission.
    b. Advise learners to speak more slowly and distinctly.
    c. Ask the learning center to develop accent reduction classes and/or modules.
    d. Develop learning contracts outlining self-improvement activities to reduce accent.

56. Some learners in the school of nursing have been found to plagiarize (intentionally or unintentionally) when writing research papers, resulting in a number of disciplinary actions. Which of the following is the best solution to prevent further plagiarism?
    a. Advise learners they will be expelled for plagiarism.
    b. Require all papers to be scanned through plagiarism detection tools.
    c. Ask learners to affirm an honor code that states they will not plagiarize.
    d. Require learners who plagiarize to write additional papers.

57. A learner who has a BE amputation of the right arm and uses a prosthetic hand has been admitted as a learner in the nursing department and will need some accommodations. Which of the following is likely to be the most effective in helping to develop modifications?
    a. Occupational therapist
    b. Rehabilitation therapist
    c. Special education instructor
    d. Physical therapist

58. A learner came to class smelling of alcohol and with slurred speech, bloodshot eyes, and hair uncombed. Which course of action should the nurse educator follow?
    a. Expel the learner from the class and recommend expulsion from the program.
    b. Tell the learner that he or she must enter a program for substance abuse to continue in the program.
    c. Ask the learner why he or she came to class in an inebriated state.
    d. Make an appointment with the learner and program director to discuss substance abuse.

59. According to Bevis (2000), which of the following is an example of *illegitimate curricula*?
    a. Knowledge and skills
    b. Caring and compassion
    c. Teaching methods
    d. Program objectives and course outlines

60. After receiving a grant from the National League for Nursing, the nurse educator and an interdisciplinary team developed a successful collaborative model for nursing education. The nurse educator believes the model would be valuable in other programs and would like to disseminate information about the model. Which of the following is the best method to share information about the model?
    a. Utilize networking to email information to contacts.
    b. Submit an article about the model to a professional journal.
    c. Give a presentation at a state and a national conference.
    d. Hold a training session at the school of nursing, mailing out flyers.

61. According to Goodland, which level of curriculum planning represents *societal curriculum*?
    a. Curriculum planned for specific populations of learners from outside the institution to standardize nursing education.
    b. Curriculum prepared by the faculty of an institution for a group of learners.
    c. Curriculum developed by an individual instructor for a particular group of learners.
    d. Curriculum proposed by learners collaborating with faculty at an institution.

62. Which of Benner's (1984) stages of clinical competence and Dreyfus and Dreyfus's (1986) model of skill acquisition likely best fit a nurse educator who has two to three years of experience and is able to cope well with job requirements but still lacks flexibility and requires extra time for planning?
    a. Advanced beginner
    b. Proficient
    c. Competent
    d. Expert

63. If a nurse educator wants to increase networking, which of the following is the best approach?
    a. Become active in professional organizations.
    b. Attend national conventions.
    c. Join professional message boards.
    d. Become active in campus committees.

64. According to Tyler, there are four primary tasks to be completed when developing curriculum. Which of the following is the first task?
    a. Select learning experiences.
    b. Organize learning experiences.
    c. Evaluate curriculum.
    d. Formulate educational objectives.

65. Which of the following educational philosophies states that curriculum should focus on problem-solving, critical thinking, and scientific research and that teachers should help learners learn how to learn rather than just teaching content?
    a. Perennialism
    b. Essentialism
    c. Progressivism
    d. Reconstructionism

66. Because of a shortage in nursing educators, the school of nursing is recruiting faculty from clinical nurse specialists and nurse practitioners employed in clinical practice. Which of the following will likely be most essential to preparing the new hires for teaching positions?
    a. Orientation to the mission and philosophy of the program.
    b. Training in learning/teaching theories and pedagogical methods.
    c. Provision of mentors for all hires for the first year.
    d. Allowing the new hires more unassigned time for independent study.

67. Which of the following is the primary impetus for the rapid changes in curriculum that are currently occurring?
    a. Changing technology
    b. Managed care
    c. Educational philosophy
    d. Increased enrollment

68. When engaged in outreach to the community to recruit new learners, the nurse educator should be aware of which three key issues facing higher education?
    a. Affordability, standardization, and globalization
    b. Affordability, access, and accountability
    c. Affordability, technology, and resources
    d. Affordability, environment, and demographic changes

69. As part of curriculum development, the nurse educator completed an extensive literature review to identify key issues and trends in nursing, healthcare, and society in order to guide curriculum development and determine future needs. Which of the following methods was the nurse educator utilizing?
    a. Forecasting: conjecture
    b. Forecasting: prediction
    c. Forecasting: projection
    d. Environmental scanning

70. The nurse educator is part of a team developing a new mission and philosophy statement for the school of nursing, but the team is having difficulty finding times when all are available to meet. Which of the following techniques of brainstorming does not require face-to-face meeting in real time?
    a. Delphi
    b. Storyboarding
    c. Critical incident/role playing
    d. Nominal group

71. The focus of outcomes assessment as part of curricular design is primarily on which of the following?
    a. Course content
    b. Learner learning
    c. Activities related to the courses
    d. Community needs

72. As part of curricular design, the nurse educator is writing the following competency statements for different levels of learners (beginning, junior, and senior nursing learners):
Develops a plan of care based on the client's goals and desired medical treatment.
Modifies a plan of care based on client's needs and outcomes.
Carries out assigned procedures for clients.

Which of the statements (numbered) are matched correctly with learner levels?

Level	a.	b.	c.	d.
Beginner	1.	2.	3	3.
Junior	2.	3.	2.	1.
Senior	3.	1.	1.	2.

73. Which of the following is an example of an active learning activity?
    a. Learner reads an assigned article
    b. Learner takes notes in class
    c. Learner watches a video presentation
    d. Learner gives an oral presentation

74. When developing curriculum outcomes, the nursing faculty has identified a number of critical learning experiences. One of these is the ability to complete a comprehensive health assessment. Which of the following is required?
    a. All learners should have practice with similar clients (age, gender).
    b. All learners should have opportunities to develop assessment skills.
    c. All learners should demonstrate skills in the same manner.
    d. All learners should have practice in similar situations (such as med-surg).

75. Which of the following are the most essential teaching behaviors (Halstead, 2002) for those teaching Internet courses?
    a. Provide rapid feedback and clearly state evaluation criteria.
    b. Establish set times for learning activities and feedback.
    c. Vary instructional methods and have synchronous office hours.
    d. Provide Internet links and a variety of resources.

76. Which of the following is an appropriate use of formative evaluation by a nurse educator teaching a course?
    a. Evaluate learner outcomes.
    b. Assess learning activities throughout a course.
    c. Determine the need for course revisions.
    d. Determine the need for clarification of material.

77. Which learning theory has the basic premise that development proceeds in a sequential manner with uneven progress through several phases?
    a. Multiple intelligences theory
    b. Cognitive learning theory
    c. Cognitive development theory
    d. Behavioral theory

78. According to information-processing theories, which component of long-term memory contains memories the person has of personal experiences?
    a. Episodic
    b. Schematic
    c. Semantic
    d. Procedural

79. When serving as a mentor to a novice nurse educator, the mentor notes that the novice educator has failed to meet the deadline for submission of course outlines. Which of the following is the best response?
    a. Remind the person that the deadline has passed.
    b. Advise the person that missing deadlines is bad policy.
    c. Tell the person to immediately turn in the course outlines.
    d. Report the person to the director of the nursing program.

80. The nurse educator is concerned that faculty does not have a strong enough voice in the faculty senate at the university. Which of the following is the best method of resolving this issue?
    a. Gather a petition of support for stronger faculty representation.
    b. Complain directly to the school of nursing and university administration.
    c. Speak to other faculty members, garnering support for a formal complaint.
    d. Run for a seat on the faculty senate in order to make changes from the inside.

81. Which of the following explains what is meant by *creating an anticipatory set* when designing learning experiences?
    a. Determining learning outcomes for a cohort of learners.
    b. Selecting teaching and learning strategies.
    c. Creating an environment that promotes learner interest.
    d. Providing an outline of course content.

82. The nurse educator must give a lecture in a 60-minute time period about nursing ethics to a group of 30 learners and is concerned that the learners remain engaged throughout the lecture. Which of the following formats presents the best option?
    a. 55-minute lecture with a 5-minute question and answer period at the end.
    b. 60-minute lecture with a post-test at the next class meeting.
    c. 50-minute lecture with a 10-minute discussion period at the end.
    d. Two 20-minute lectures with 10 minutes of discussion after each lecture.

83. Which of the following is an essential element when the nurse educator is using adult learning principles to work with adult learners?
    a. Collaboration
    b. Direction
    c. Assisted learning
    d. Prompting

84. Which of the following interpretive pedagogies is used to describe the human experience?
    a. Post-modern discourse
    b. Phenomenology
    c. Feminist pedagogy
    d. Critical pedagogy

85. Considering learner misconduct, which of the following would be classified as an administrative violation rather than criminal conduct or an annoying act?
    a. Refusing to cooperate with the instructor during a class exercise.
    b. Hitting another class member during a disagreement.
    c. Cheating on a test.
    d. Repeatedly texting someone during the class period.

86. As a teaching strategy, the use of games in class is most appropriate for which of the following?
    a. Introduction of new concepts
    b. Knowledge reinforcement
    c. Skills instruction
    d. Tension reduction

87. During a role-playing activity, one participant becomes extremely upset and begins yelling inappropriately at the other participant. Which of the following is the best response for the nurse educator?

    a. Suspend the role playing and initiate a discussion about the reaction.

    b. Stop the role-playing activity altogether.

    c. Continue the role-playing to see if the participants can resolve the issue.

    d. Replace the participant who is upset and continue the role-playing.

88. A novice nurse educator gives a test of 100 multiple-choice questions to a group of 15 learners. The resultant scores are distributed as follows: 90, 86, 82, 79, 79, 74, 72, 71, 69, 64, 62, 62, 55, 54, and 40.

After the learners complain that they had difficulty understanding the questions, the nurse educator reviews the test with a more experienced teacher and finds that some questions are ambiguous and some are too difficult. Because of this, the nurse educator must make a decision about the type of grading. Which of the following is likely the best solution:

a.	b.	c.	d.
Absolute 10%	Relative, 10%	Relative, grouped	No grade
A = 90 B = 86, 82 C = 79, 74, 72, 71 D = 69, 64, 62 F = 55, 54, 40	A = 90, 86, 82 B = 79,74 C = 72, 72, 69, 64 D = 62, 55 F = 54, 40	A = 90, 86 B = 82, 79 C = 74, 72, 71, 69 D = 64, 62 F = 55, 54, 40	Discard test

89. A nurse educator plans to use a classroom assessment technique (CAT) at the end of each class to determine if the learners are able to identify the most important issues covered in a series of classes about critical thinking. Which of the following is likely the best choice?

    a. Multiple-choice questionnaire

    b. 5-minute discussion period

    c. True/false questionnaire

    d. One-minute essay

90. A nurse educator believes that the learners do not have enough exposure to multicultural content and plans to incorporate multicultural perspectives into the classes. Which of the following is likely to be most beneficial for learners?

    a. Guest speakers from different cultures discussing cultural/health attitudes.

    b. A series of videos about different cultural groups and healthcare.

    c. Readings about multicultural attitudes related to life and health.

    d. Field trips to a variety of ethnic communities for observation.

91. The school of nursing has admitted a group of foreign learners from Asian countries. The nurse educator finds that these learners are more accustomed to education by lecture and are more comfortable as passive learners, but the teaching strategies require active participation. The nurse educator has explained the difference in classroom dynamics in the United States and Asian countries, but this has not changed behavior. Which of the following is the best approach to dealing with this issue?

    a. Change to a lecture format for all classroom presentations.

    b. Develop structural small group exercises to facilitate interaction.

    c. Tell learners that they will fail the class if they do not participate.

    d. Advise the administration against enrolling further foreign learners.

92. The three criteria required for cultural competence include *knowledge, skills,* and which of the following?

    a. Attitudes

    b. Tolerance

    c. Patience

    d. Acceptance

93. As part of a program focusing on breast cancer prevention, the local health department is partnering with the school of nursing to train learners to do breast exams utilizing a standardized client who has been trained to undergo the exams for nurses and physicians and comment on the learners' techniques. While the standardized client is aware that some learners are male and does not object, some of the male learners have expressed concern to the nurse educator about doing a breast exam. Which of the following is the most appropriate solution by the nurse educator?

    a. Discuss the issue of inappropriate touching vs. medical examination.

    b. Allow male learners who are concerned to opt out of the training.

    c. Tell the male learners that they must participate in the training.

    d. Allow the male learners to practice breast exams with a simulator.

94. A nurse educator is a clinical instructor for learners in orthopedics. Which of the following attributes are most important for the clinical instructor?

    a. Patience and empathy

    b. Knowledge and patience

    c. Clinical skills and judgment

    d. Patience and kindness

95. In a small group post-clinical conference, a learner undergoing a clinical rotation on a post-surgical orthopedic unit admits that when a client expressed concern that he would be crippled after surgical repair of traumatic injuries related to an automobile accident, the learner, realizing this was true but not knowing how to respond, made a joke and left the room. What is the best response of the nurse educator?

    a. "That was a very poor response to the client's concerns."
    b. "In retrospect, how would you respond differently?"
    c. "How would you rate that response to the client?"
    d. "Don't feel bad. Everyone makes these kinds of mistakes."

96. Which of the following is the first thing a clinical nurse instructor must do before instituting nursing rounds with a client?

    a. Provide information about the client to the learners.
    b. Prepare a series of questions to serve as a guide.
    c. Ask permission of the client's physician.
    d. Gain permission from the client for nursing rounds.

97. The nurse educator is considering the use of the paired model for the learner's clinical experience. Which of the following does this model entail?

    a. The learner will be assigned a preceptor.
    b. The learner will be paired with a staff nurse.
    c. A staff nurse will conduct a small group of learners.
    d. Two learners will work together as a team.

98. The nurse educator wants the learners to do a written self-evaluation at the end of the clinical experience. Which is the best method to assist the learners to develop the skills needed to evaluate themselves effectively?

    a. Ask learners to informally evaluate their performances on a regular basis.
    b. Provide an example of a self-evaluation done by an earlier learner.
    c. Explain in detail what is expected in self-evaluations.
    d. Guide learners through the self-evaluation, one-on-one.

99. Which of the following is the most important factor when the nurse educator is selecting a preceptor to work with a particular learner in the clinical environment?

    a. The preceptor wants to work with learners.
    b. The preceptor has previous experience working with learners.
    c. The preceptor communicates freely with the nurse educator.
    d. The preceptor has many years of experience in nursing.

100. Which of the following best describes a clinical teaching partnership?
    a. The nurse educator works in conjunction with a clinical nurse specialist at the facility, guiding and supervising learners through clinical experience.
    b. The nurse educator assigns a clinical nurse specialist to work with a group of learners and to provide formative evaluations in order to improve clinical skills.
    c. The nurse educator, who is a full-time faculty member, works half time at the school of nursing and half time at the facility, guiding and supervising learners.
    d. The nurse educator schedules clinical experiences but a clinical nurse specialist at the facility serving as an adjunct does clinical assignments and supervision.

101. Considering psychomotor skill categories (Alavi et al., 1991), the nurse educator is aware that it is more difficult to obtain learner practice in skills classified as *specialized* therapeutic and diagnostic skills as opposed to *fundamental* or *general* skills. Which of the following skills is least likely to be readily available for learners to practice as part of clinical experience?
    a. Lifting and transferring clients
    b. Inserting a nasogastric tube
    c. Administering IV therapy
    d. Changing surgical dressings

102. Before implementing a simulation in the learning lab in which a patient in the ICU experiences respiratory failure, the nurse educator should complete which of the following?
    a. A checklist of required learner actions
    b. A guide for learners that specifies required actions
    c. Practice of the scenario to pinpoint necessary timing
    d. A pretest for the learners to assess knowledge base

103. The nurse educator has written the following essay question:
    Compare Orlando's nursing process theory, Hoff's crisis theory of nursing, and Benner's stages of clinical competence with each other and describe both similarities and differences. Then, utilizing aspects from each of these theories, develop a personal theory of nursing.

When developing an analytic scoring rubric worksheet for grading the essay response, what is the minimum number of separate items that should be analyzed for scoring?
    a. Two
    b. Four
    c. Five
    d. Nine

104. Which term describes the observational learning effect of one learner observing another learner behave in a manner in class that is socially unacceptable, such as ignoring the instructor and talking on a cellphone, when that behavior is tolerated and the first learner suffers no consequences?
a. Inhibition
b. Facilitation
c. Imitation
d. Disinhibition

105. In order to ensure that learners encode information into long-term memory, the nurse educator must include which of the following in lesson plans?
a. Explanations of the importance of learning.
b. Frequent pre- and post-tests.
c. Opportunities to review and rehearse.
d. Instruction regarding short-term and long-term memory.

106. Which of the following do learners experience when observing behavior from the nurse educator that models their own behavior and teaches that they are successful because of past success?
a. Self-determination
b. Self-actualization
c. Self-efficacy
d. Self-fulfillment

107. Which of the following is a key belief of the social reform perspective of teaching?
a. Learning entails a search for meaning, influenced by prior knowledge.
b. Content should be learned in its authorized form and taught by experts.
c. Knowledge is best acquired in the environment in which it will be used.
d. Knowledge contains values and beliefs that must be examined.

108. The school of nursing has been presenting a number of free classes about general and specific health conditions for community members but after the current fiscal year (and one more semester) must discontinue the program because of cost-cutting measures related to decreased state funding of the university. Which of the following alternatives is the best solution?
a. Decrease class offering during the final semester and divert funds to develop free interactive Internet classes.
b. Continue with the classes for the final semester and then discontinue the program.
c. Discontinue the classes immediately and divert funds to other uses.
d. Continue the program indefinitely and rely on volunteer nurse educators to teach the classes.

109. The school of nursing is located near a large immigrant Hispanic community, which has an approximate 12% rate of diabetes among adults. Many adults remain undiagnosed and untreated, resulting in frequent emergency department visits and hospitalizations. The nurse educator would like to utilize service learning to target this problem. Which of the following options may provide the best service to the community?

    a. Groups of learners are sent each week to volunteer at a free clinic that provides diabetes testing and diabetic medications to members of the community.

    b. Groups of learners set up diabetic screening and information booths (with translators) throughout the community in parks, churches, malls, and community centers.

    c. Learners develop informational handouts about diabetes (translated into Spanish) to distribute throughout the community.

    d. Groups of learners attend political meetings in the community to stress the need for increased diagnosis and treatment of diabetes.

110. The nurse educator notes that learners undergoing practice with physical assessment utilizing simulated clients have the most difficulty assessing cardiac and respiratory sounds, but learners are limited in the time they can spend practicing because there is only one simulator for a large group of learners. Which of the following solutions should the nurse educator consider?

    a. Provide additional literature about normal and abnormal cardiac and respiratory sounds.

    b. Have the learners practice assessing cardiac and respiratory sounds with each other.

    c. Have groups of learners assess hospitalized clients with abnormal cardiac or respiratory sounds.

    d. Provide an interactive Internet or CD-ROM program that provides examples of abnormal cardiac and respiratory sounds.

111. The nurse educator has videotaped a role-playing exercise in which the learners interview a community volunteer who is playing the role of a client. One learner is very nervous during the exercise, continually rubbing the hands together, licking lips, and stuttering when interviewing the "client." Which of the following is the best response for the nurse educator when viewing the videotape with the learner?

    a. "I can see that you were very nervous."

    b. "Let's talk about ways you can control your nervousness."

    c. "What do you see when you watch your interaction with the client?"

    d. "What can you do to be more relaxed during an interview with a client?"

112. The nurse educator would like to arrange for a guest speaker to address the learners, but the speaker works at a different university and cannot take time off to come to the school of nursing. Which of the following is the best solution?
    a. Get a different guest speaker with similar knowledge and background.
    b. Utilize videoconferencing to allow the speaker to address the learners.
    c. Show a videotape of the speaker from a conference presentation.
    d. Have learners use a Web-based interactive program produced by the speaker.

113. If the nurse educator administers the same test on two different occasions to the same group of learners and finds that the results are almost the same, the test has which of the following?
    a. Reliability
    b. Validity
    c. Accessibility
    d. Reproducibility

114. The nurse educator is writing an assessment instrument for a nursing course. Which of the following is required to validate the instrument?
    a. Trial administration
    b. Review by other instructors
    c. High reliability
    d. Evidence

115. When the nurse educator administers a test to a group of learners, they point out that the questions do not appear to relate to the content studied in the class. Which of the following does the test appear to lack?
    a. Reliability
    b. Generalizability
    c. Face validity
    d. Validity

116. When developing test items, each item should be designed primarily to test mastery of which of the following?
    a. Course content
    b. Course objectives
    c. Clinical skills
    d. Learning outcomes

117. The nurse educator plans to develop a series of test items for a unit of study. Which of the following test items is a *constructed-response* type?
    a. Multiple-choice
    b. Completion
    c. Matching
    d. True/False

118. During the first semester of teaching, the nurse educator provided a personal email address to learners and encouraged them to contact her at any time, promising that she would respond within two to four hours; however, she found she was receiving a large number of emails at all hours and often with trivial questions or comments. The nurse educator is reconsidering this approach for the second semester. Which of the following is the best solution?
    a. Continue with the same but advise learners to limit emails to questions.
    b. Discontinue emails and tell learners to contact her during office hours.
    c. Provide an email address for emergency use only.
    d. Set email "office hours" during which the nurse educator will respond.

119. The nurse educator is preparing a blueprint worksheet for an exam covering the first two units of a textbook but has not yet completed the worksheet. The course has four objectives, which are weighted according to importance. There will be 100 questions on the test:

	Total items	Obj. 1-40%	Obj. 2-30%	Obj. 3-20%	Obj. 4-10%
Unit 1	60	24		12	
Unit 2		16			4

Based on this blueprint, how many test items should be assigned for Unit 2, Objective 2?
    a. 12
    b. 16
    c. 18
    d. 24

120. When developing a true/false test, what is the maximum number of repeats of the same answer (true or false) that the nurse educator should use in a sequence of answers?
    a. Two
    b. Three
    c. Four
    d. Five

121. Which is the most effective method of preventing cheating among learners?
    a. Assign seats different from usual seating.
    b. Warn learners of punishment for cheating.
    c. Remind learners of moral code.
    d. Give each learner a different test.

122. The nurse educator has utilized a computer software program to assess internal consistency and the reliability coefficient of four different forms (A, B, C, and D) of a test. Based on the reliability coefficients, which of the following tests has the most reliability?

    a. 1.0

    b. 0.8

    c. 0.4

    d. 0.0

123. The school of nursing is considering modifying admission policies, which are currently based on grade point averages. Grade inflation has limited the value of transcripts in determining if a learner is qualified for admission, with many learners requiring remediation in math and English. Which of the following is likely the best choice for an initial additional measure?

    a. SAT scores

    b. Personal interview

    c. Nursing aptitude test

    d. Basic skills test

124. Despite discussing deficiencies with a senior in the nursing program, establishing a learning contract to allow the learner to meet required standards, and assigning a mentor to guide the learner, the learner, who has good grades in testing, consistently fails to meet standards in clinical evaluations, often putting clients at risk because of failure to follow through on basic nursing care and assessment. Which is the best solution when assigning the learner a grade at the end of the term, at which time the learner is due to graduate?

    a. Pass the learner based on testing scores.

    b. Suggest the learner take a leave of absence.

    c. Assign the learner a failing grade.

    d. Recommend the learner retake the senior year.

125. During a class of professional standards, the nurse educator discusses his thoughts about his own educational experiences and educational needs, describing the strengths and weaknesses of his education, his academic performance, his attitudes toward education, and his future educational needs as a professional. Which of the following types of thinking is the nurse educator modeling?

    a. Reflective thinking

    b. Critical thinking

    c. Lateral thinking

    d. Strategic thinking

126. The nurse educator uses brief evaluations by learners at the end of each class session to determine what is effective and what is less effective in order to modify course content. Which of the following does this action on the part of the nurse educator primarily represent?

    a. Continuous quality improvement.
    b. Empowerment of learners to bring about change.
    c. Insecurity regarding course content.
    d. Exercise in professional ethics.

127. When conducting a detailed item analysis of multiple-choice questions, the nurse educator finds the following P values and point biserial index (PBI) (correct answer noted beside question number and bolded):

Choices	Question 1 – C		Question 2 -B		Question 3 – A		Question 4 -D	
	P	PBI	P	PBI	P	PBI	P	PBI
A	0.72	-0.46	0.26	- 0.62	0.35	0.50	0.69	-0.16
B		-0.28		-0.14		-0.25		-0.23
C		0.43		0.24		-0.04		-0.19
D		-0.30		0.041		-0.28		0.28

Based on these values, which of the questions does the nurse educator need to discard or rewrite?

    a. Question 1
    b. Question 2
    c. Question 3
    d. Question 4

128. The nurse educator finds that scores on one exam were significantly lower than for other exams and feels that the scores on this exam will negatively affect the learners' final grades and progression to the next level. Which of the following is the best solution?

    a. Assign grades according to scores earned on the exam.
    b. Discard the exam and the learners' score.
    c. Allow learners to complete an extra credit project.
    d. Assign an additional test so learners have more overall points.

129. The NCLEX-RN pass rate for the nursing program dropped from 95% to 87% with the last group of graduates. Which of the following is the best beginning point for evaluating the reason for this decline?

    a. Internal surveys and interviews with faculty and current learners.
    b. Follow-up surveys and interviews with those taking the NCLEX exam.
    c. Review of compliance with accreditation standards.
    d. Review of NCLEX group-performance data.

130. As part of program evaluation, the school of nursing plans to conduct surveys to determine how well graduates have done post-graduation. Which of the following is the best initial approach?

    a. Conduct Internet surveys of graduates and employers 6 to 12 months after graduation.

    b. Conduct telephone interviews with graduates 3 to 6 months after graduation.

    c. Send out printed surveys to nursing employers with no regard to time since graduation.

    d. Conduct one-on-one interviews with locally-employed graduates 6 months to 4 years after graduation.

131. In order to evaluate satisfaction with the nursing program by current learners, the faculty members of the school of nursing have conducted personal interviews and surveys with all learners during their evaluations. How should the results of this information be presented to the program directors and board?

    a. As individual and compiled group data

    b. As individual data only

    c. As compiled group data

    d. As a narrative summary of data

132. Which of the following is a primary component of Freire's (1970) theory of emancipatory education?

    a. Scholarship

    b. Outcomes

    c. Discipline

    d. Reflection

133. The nurse educator has proposed that the nursing program include a course on nursing informatics and the director of the program has asked the nurse educator to develop a sample outline of possible course content before the proposed course is considered. Which of the following is the best method of developing the outline?

    a. Copy an outline from another university offering such a course.

    b. Obtain copies of course outlines from a number of universities.

    c. Take an Internet course in nursing informatics to determine the best content.

    d. Conduct research about nursing informatics on databases and in the library.

134. During clinical rotations, the clinical nurse educator received complaints from a number of clients about learners' communication skills and feels that more attention needs to be paid to communicating with clients. Which of the following is the best method to promote better communication skills and to evaluate them?

    a. Accompany learners to client's rooms to observe communications.

    b. Conduct surveys with clients about the learners' communication skills.

    c. Conduct additional role-playing exercises for learners.

    d. Assign process recordings to learners as a form of self-evaluation.

135. The nurse educator is concerned that an educationally-disadvantaged learner is at risk for failure despite support programs because of poor academic performance and unsatisfactory clinical competencies. Which of the following is the best approach to dealing with this issue?

    a. Provide the learner formative evaluations and remedial work.

    b. Advise the learner that progress is unsatisfactory.

    c. Notify the administration that the learner may fail.

    d. Suggest the learner transfer out of the nursing program.

136. According to Chen's (1990) theory-driven program evaluation and normative outcome evaluation, *goal realizability evaluations* do which of the following?

    a. Identify desired goals and outcomes for the program.

    b. Prioritize goals and outcomes according to the importance given by stakeholders.

    c. Assess consistency between program goals and activities.

    d. Compare and contrast program goals with the organizational mission.

137. Which of the following is a linear theory that explains changes in behavior in terms of a threat, which serves as a stimulus to develop coping appraisal and behavior change?

    a. Reasoned action

    b. Stages of change (Transtheoretical)

    c. Self-efficacy

    d. Protection motivation

138. The nurse educator is working with an interdisciplinary group to develop an outreach program for the community, but some members complain that others are too critical of their contributions. In order to maintain a productive but positive working environment, what ratio of compliments to criticism should the members strive for?

    a. 1:1

    b. 2:1

    c. 3:1

    d. 4:1

139. With the support of the state board of nursing and professional nursing organizations, a legislator has proposed legislation requiring minimum client-to-staff ratios in acute hospitals in the state. The nurse educator would like to support this effort. Which of the following methods of support is likely to be the most effective?

    a. Vote in every state election to support those in favor of the proposal.

    b. Participate actively in professional organizations at the state level.

    c. Visit members of the legislature personally to ask for support.

    d. Write letters to legislators in support of the legislation.

140. Which is the first step in facilitating change within an organization?
   a. Deciding on the steps to facilitate change.
   b. Taking action to bring about change.
   c. Developing an understanding of the change process.
   d. Believing that change is possible.

141. The school of nursing had established a goal of increasing the NCLEX pass rate from 86% to 90%, but the pass rate increased from 86% to 92%. Which of the following is the best response?
   a. Reward the faculty for hard work and dedication.
   b. Advertise the results as part of marketing for the school.
   c. Send letters of congratulation to the learners who passed the NCLEX.
   d. Research the results to determine what increased the pass rate.

142. Following submission of an article about an innovative program at the school of nursing to a journal and acceptance for publication, the nurse educator finds evidence that one of the internal studies that was used had significant errors in calculations although these did not change the ultimate outcomes. Which is the most appropriate action?
   a. Take no action as the faulty calculations do not affect outcomes.
   b. Immediately notify the journal of inaccuracies in content.
   c. Ask for advice about proceeding from the director of nursing.
   d. Allow publication but write an explanation for the following issue.

143. When designing successful Web-based instruction, which of the following is the key factor?
   a. Security
   b. Collaborative learning opportunities
   c. Interactivity
   d. Cost-effectiveness

144. The nurse educator is not in a position of management but has been urged by the nursing director to take a leadership course. Which of the following is the best reason for the nurse educator to develop leadership skills?
   a. The nurse educator may advance into a management position.
   b. The nurse educator interacts with and influences learners and professionals.
   c. The nurse educator will gain a better understanding of management.
   d. The nurse educator will have increased job satisfaction.

145. Which of the following teaching perspectives is based on the premise that learning requires both cognitive and affective processes and is impaired by anxiety and threats to self-esteem?
    a. Nurturing
    b. Apprenticeship
    c. Development
    d. Transmission

146. In context-based learning, after the learners have been presented with a situation that is examined and learning issues and information sources have been identified, what is the next phase in the process for the learners?
    a. Formulate learning objectives and outcome goals.
    b. Gather information and study independently or in a group.
    c. Reflect on the context and the learning process.
    d. Discuss information and apply it the situation.

147. Which of the following groups is most responsible for identifying opportunities for improvement in healthcare?
    a. Administrators
    b. Politicians
    c. Everyone
    d. Educators

148. The nurse educator is reviewing the documentation of a learner describing observations of a client. Which of the following statements best describes the observation in non-biased terms?
    a. "The client stayed in her room with the lights out and did not respond to questions."
    b. "The client was depressed and non-responsive."
    c. "The client withdrew from association with others and rejected interactions."
    d. "The client was visibly upset and refused to answer questions."

149. When completing a learning contract with a learner, the nurse educator must ensure that the four major components of the learning contract are included. The four components are *content, performance expectations, evaluation,* and which of the following?
    a. Resources
    b. Time frame
    c. Purpose
    d. Processes

150. Which of the following addresses the *conservative principle* (Aggarwal) of curriculum development?

 a. Provide a foundation of knowledge.

 b. Plan according to activity and experience.

 c. Discard topics and activities no longer required by current learners.

 d. Provide flexibility rather than rigidity in curriculum development.

Answers and Explanations

1. B: When the nurse educator is preparing a lesson regarding culturally-sensitive care, the nurse should begin with examining and considering personal culture because the nurse educator first needs to understand his or her own perceptions and biases. Nursing education tends to be Eurocentric, even though Eurocentric beliefs and values may not represent those of learners from different cultures. Nurse educators may exhibit cultural bias when utilizing teaching strategies that are more appropriate for some cultures than for others.

2. D: There are many reasons why learners choose an AS program. AS programs are often more flexible and allow part-time enrollment, they may be nearer to people's homes, and they are often less expensive than BSN programs, so choosing a BSN program may not be realistic. However, the nurse educator should tell learners that they should consider taking an RN-to-BSN bridge program. In many states, distance-learning plans are available for the bridge programs, and some employers provide tuition assistance.

3. A: The best solution for a learner with a high threat perception that has resulted in the learner being too frightened to adequately provide care to clients in a clinical rotation is to assign the learner to work with a preceptor. The learner can work with the preceptor under guidance without the fear of being responsible for the client and doing harm. A reflective journal is a good exercise, but removing the learner from the clinical rotation may not be possible, and a nurse educator with a number of students to monitor cannot accompany one learner.

4. B: When the nurse educator is in a position of leadership and must meet with a staff member to discuss inadequate performance, the first step is to describe the behavior that requires change. Then, the nurse educator should explain how the person's behavior is affecting staff attitudes and performance. Next, the nurse educator should outline the steps that the staff member needs to take to make necessary changes and advise the person of the consequences for failure to make the changes.

5. A: Computer-based training (CBT) can be used to provide or support course content. Advantages are that the training is self-paced, allowing the individual flexibility in the speed of learning, and there may be access to the course for 24 hours a day, especially if it is Internet-based. Training can be offered online and offline. CBT improves retention, especially when it involves interactivity and is used to teach about technology, such as in the course "Information and Technology Literacy," and facilitates mastery by allowing learners to review and progress as they are able.

6. D: While it may be tempting to offer materials or give suggestions to a novice instructor, the best response is to ask the novice nurse if the experienced nurse can be of assistance in some way, leaving it to the novice nurse to decide. It is normal for a novice nurse to require more time to develop course content and materials because of a lack of experience. It is good to empathize, but if the experienced nurse only empathizes, the novice nurse may not feel comfortable asking for needed assistance.

7. B: When plotting learner scores on a Bell curve, the nurse educator expects that 68% of the scores will fall within one standard deviation of the mean while 95% will fall within two standard deviations of the mean and >99% within 3 standard deviations of the mean. If the number of scores within the first standard deviation falls, then this usually means that the test was too easy (if the scores skew higher) or too hard (if the scores skew lower).

8. C: The first thing the nurse educator should do before beginning the application process for a federal grant is to read through a number of successful grant applications. For example, the Health Resources and Services Administration provides abstracts and contact information for those who have received grants; and most colleges and universities have received grants at some point, and these should be available. Once familiar with the process, the nurse educator should carefully read through the directions for the application, noting dates of deadlines, before proceeding further.

9. A: According to the National League for Nursing's *Excellence in Nursing Education Model©*, a "well-prepared faculty" is comprised of members with expertise in different areas, rather than faculty comprising all researchers or all expert clinicians. The needs of nursing education are varied, although all should be focused on excellence in teaching. Expert clinicians are needed to guide clinical practice and develop evidenced-based teaching while researchers and academic scholars are needed for such activities as guiding curriculum development and writing grants.

10. D: According to the Kolb Learning Style Inventory, the type of learning experience the learner with an assimilative style likely prefers is abstract conceptualization and reflective observation. This type of learner enjoys working with abstract concepts, analyzing ideas systematically; they are often able to consider ideas and situations impartially and consider many points of view. These learners are often engaged in the fields of math and science, such as physics, and they enjoy research.

11. C: A commitment to lifelong learning is exemplified by consistently seeking information, such as the nurse educator who reads professional journals and is taking an Internet course. Vague future plans only count if they come to fruition; and while there is value in attending a conference, lifelong learning requires more than an annual commitment in time. Continuing education courses that are required for

licensure don't reflect commitment to learning so much as commitment to maintaining professional licensure.

12. A: Socialization in the role of nurse educator refers to socialization related primarily to the nurse educator's professional (as opposed to personal or social) role, so the best activity to promote socialization would be to participate in meetings, committees, and other professional activities. These types of activities help the nurse educator to network, to meet other people in the field, to share ideas with fellow professionals, and to learn from others. Additionally, the nurse educator can gain a wide variety of experiences and increased knowledge.

13. C: Because some women feel uncomfortable with male nurses caring for them in obstetrics (even though many of the physicians are male), the best solution for the nurse educator is to specifically ask clients if they are comfortable with a male nurse. This avoids placing the male learners in the position of being rejected and also saves the time required to reassign the learners when a client refuses care. The nurse educator also has an opportunity to educate clients about the importance of males in nursing and to encourage acceptance.

14. C: 20. Total test items = 50:

	Unit 1	Unit 2
Lecture hours	10	6
% of lecture hours	60%	40%
Number of exam items	30	20

Generally, when determining how many test items to write for each unit, a range of numbers is indicated, such as 28 to 32 instead of 30, and 18 to 22 instead of 20, to allow for variations in content. The number of items should reflect the degree of emphasis of the material in the class and the class time spent studying the material.

15. B: Cultural relativism: People's beliefs and practices can only be accurately judged from within the context of their own cultures. Ethnocentrism: People's belief that their culture and way of thinking and living is the only one that is right and that those who differ are in error. Cultural competence: People's conscious awareness of their own cultures and ability to use this knowledge to avoid influencing those from other cultures. Cultural awareness: People's ability to recognize and appreciate the culture of others.

16. A: When a nurse educator wants to make substantive changes to the nursing program, the educator must follow standard procedures, recognizing the hierarchical structure of the organization and avoiding antagonizing those who may be needed for support. Any proposed changes should first be discussed with the director of the school of nursing, who may be aware of issues (such as financing) to which the nurse educator is not aware and, if receptive, may be able to provide invaluable guidance.

17. C: In story-based learning, *letting learn* refers to allowing learners to go through required content to determine what information is needed rather than the educator identifying behavioral objectives. The goal is for learners to acquire knowledge for purpose rather than just for them to memorize facts. Story-based learning is based on both case-method teaching and problem-based learning, so it promotes self-directed learning with learner-centered education.

18. D: When a test has multiple types of questions, the questions should be grouped by type so that each type can be preceded by one explanation. It is better to scramble questions than to group them by content. The educator should avoid repeating the same letter for answers more than 2 or 3 times in a row and avoid patterns of answers, as learners may use these patterns to guess answers. Usually, questions that are easier or that require less time to answer are grouped first and time-consuming questions, such as essay questions, are placed last.

19. A: Using the PSCOT method, the nurse educator would outline the question (Would graduating nurses who participated in the mentoring program have higher NCLEX scores than those who participated in NCLEX workshops during their last semester?) as follows:
Population: Graduating nurses
Strategy: Mentoring
Comparison: NCLEX workshops
Outcomes: NCLEX score
Time: Last semester

The PSCOT method can be used with any population—learners, educators, administrators, and clients. In some cases, time may be omitted if it is not an important factor.

20. C: While compensation, job security, and congenial environment are important factors for job satisfaction, the primary factor is the opportunity to advance, such as through promotion or more responsibilities. People often become frustrated in "dead end" jobs with no hope for advancement and may look elsewhere for employment, so any work environment should allow for growth and development, even if it only means the authority to make changes in the current role while remaining at the same level of employment.

21. A: Informational empowerment is derived from sharing useful information, such as that from research and Internet searches, with peers, or others. This type of empowerment is especially valuable in an organization. Referent empowerment is derived from affiliating with other members of the organization who have positions of power. Rewarding empowerment is derived from the ability to give recognition and rewards to others in the organization. Connecting empowerment is derived from working closely or having a mentoring relationship with a person in authority.

22. D: The best approach to teaching a psychomotor skill is to focus only on the steps to carrying out the skill, because learning psychomotor skills requires full concentration, and interjecting questions or discussion may interfere with the learning process. Discussion of principles is directed at the cognitive domain and usually precedes instruction of the psychomotor skill to prepare the learners. Discussing feelings is part of the affective domain and may be done before and/or after instruction of the psychomotor skill.

23. B: CINAHL (Cumulative Index to Nursing and Allied Health Literature), available via EBSCOhost, is the most useful resource for nurse educators researching evidence-based teaching strategies because it indexes articles about nursing education. Different versions of the database are available. CINAHL contains millions of articles (from 1981), indexes more than 3000 journals, and has full text of more than 70 journals. CINAHL Plus, Plus with Full Text, and Complete index from 1937. The MEDLINE database is also useful.

24. A: Analysis. Levels of cognitive behavior:
Knowledge: Able to memorize and learn facts, rules, principles, and terms.
Comprehension: Able to define or explain in own words.
Application: Able to use information in specific situations.
Analysis: Able to recognize and use information by seeing a relationship.
Synthesis: Able to take parts and create a unified whole.
Evaluation: Able to judge the value of information.

25. D: The primary purpose of a curriculum philosophy statement, which is a statement of values and beliefs about education, is to guide the development of curriculum, helping educators make decisions about content, strategies, and sequencing. Philosophy statements do not outline actions but should be compatible with the philosophy of the institution and congruent with actual education practice. In some institutions, learning theories, which are based on both theory and philosophy, are used in place of curriculum philosophy.

26. C: The Synergy Model, when applied to education, assigns descriptors to learners. Resilience is the learner characteristic that refers to the learner's adaptability to differences in teaching styles and strategies and different styles of learning. Readiness is a state of being prepared and motivated to learn. Vulnerability is the degree to which learners react to real or potential stressors. Predictability is the degree to which learning is expected.

27. B: While the clinical instructor may be involved in all of these roles to some degree, the primary role should be guiding learners and facilitating learning through the development of learning activities that are appropriate for the learners and the context. The clinical instructor's actions may be focused on teaching, but this should

always be done from the perspective of guidance in order to support and motivate learners and help them to become self-directed learners.

28. A: According to Boyer, faculty members engage in different types of scholarship: discovery, integration, application, and teaching. The scholarship of discovery refers to conducting original research or developing new knowledge and is considered the foundation for the other types of scholarship because discovery provides the knowledge base. The scholarship of discovery is utilized when developing evidence-based practice. Federal grant money is often awarded for those involved in scholarship of discovery, and some tenure decisions are also based on this type of scholarship.

29. D: Competency statements are developed after desired program outcomes and require consideration of the right learner, the right behavior, and the right context:
Right learner: This should clearly describe the type and level of learner, such as freshman nursing learner or pre-nursing learner.
Right behavior: This should describe the level of performance expected for this learner.
Right context: This should describe the particular environment in which the learner is expected to demonstrate the appropriate level of performance.

30. A: The principle of *vertical organization* refers to the reasons behind sequencing of courses based on elements of the curriculum, which should increase in complexity and level of difficulty. During evaluation, the reviewers should determine if course objectives reflect this increase in complexity and level of difficulty throughout the sequence of courses. Other principles are those of *internal consistency*, which looks at curricular design in terms of objectives, subject matter, activities and outcomes; and *linear congruence/horizontal organization,* which guides course placement in terms of preceding, following, or taking concurrently.

31. C: MeSH (Medical Subject Headings) is a vocabulary used to index materials on PubMed and some other health databases (CINAHL) and to serve as a thesaurus for searching on those databases. MeSH contains coded subject headings (C, for example, represents diseases), also referred to as descriptors, arranged in a hierarchical manner with subheadings. Subject headings may contain descriptions (brief). MeSH also provides a list of standard qualifiers that can be added to descriptors to narrow search parameters.

32. C: Confidence. Keller's (1987) ARCS model for creating a motivating learning environment includes:
Attention: Case studies, comparisons, opposing ideas, variable teaching strategies. Gaining attention may be done by perceptual arousal (surprise, uncertainty) or inquiry arousal (questioning).
Relevance: Learners' experience, usefulness (current and future), matching personal needs, and choices.

Confidence: Learning requirements, difficulty level, learner expectations, and sense of accomplishment.

Satisfaction: Timely utilization of new skills, rewards, praise (while avoiding patronizing the learner by over-rewarding), and self-evaluation.

33. B: Assessing learners at the beginning of each class for learning styles and learning needs supports the National League for Nursing's Nurse Educator Competencies related to facilitating learner development and socialization. Other supporting methods include providing resources, counseling, recognizing how learning and teaching styles relate to outcomes, and modeling professional behavior. Additionally, the nurse educator should create learning environments that focus on socialization to help learners understand the role of nurses and to set personal goals.

34. C: While the traditional learners often can attend nursing school fulltime during the day, increasingly, this schedule is difficult for people with low income to manage because many low-paying jobs are more common during the daytime, and daycare for young children may be a problem as well. The best solution for the school is to offer classes in the evening and online and to allow part-time admission so that people who are working can take longer to complete their coursework.

35. A: Algorithms are most useful when teaching skills that involve a number of steps and "yes-no" decisions regarding actions, such as "Is there redness about the site?" leading to two different options depending on whether the answer is "yes" or "no."

It can take up to 8 hours to develop an effective algorithm, so this is an instructor-intensive teaching method, but associated algorithms may require less investment of time. The steps must be very clear to enable learners to complete tasks accurately.

36. D: A nurse educator who has a good sense of humor, cares about learners, and serves as a mentor is exhibiting competencies related to relationships with learners and colleagues. Other attributes include acting as a role model, showing respect for others, being accepting of cultural and ethnic diversity, and providing a supportive atmosphere in which others—both learners and colleagues—can feel safe and flourish. The competent nurse serves as an advocate for learners and assists them through advisement and counseling.

37. B: Debates are most effective for issues in which there is a clear ethical dilemma or controversy because evidence is usually available that supports both sides, making for a more interesting debate and easier access to supporting evidence. In this case, the best topic is "assisted suicide for the terminally ill." Debating helps learners develop skills in analysis and may help them to consider alternative ways of thinking, but the debate format is foreign to many learners, so teaching the art of debate may be time consuming.

38. C: The type of bias evident when appropriate health information related to an ethnic minority is not included in a textbook is omission/invisibility. Other types of biases found in instructional materials include stereotyping, imbalance or selectivity in which some information is included but other important information is excluded, fragmentation and isolation, and linguistic bias. The nurse educator should review instructional materials for these types of biases and should utilize other materials or supplement materials as needed to compensate.

39. D: The characteristics of Millennials/Generation Y (born 1981 to 2003) include being optimistic, socially aware, direct, vocal, and socially involved. This generation tends to follow rules and they are good team players as they have grown up during a time when teamwork has been stressed. Generation Y tends to be comfortable with technology, as members have always had computers and other electronic and digital equipment and feel connection to the Internet is essential. Generation Y is more diverse than previous generations with over a third being non-white or Hispanic.

40. A: The nurse educator might expect that a learner who shows a preference for introversion over extroversion in the Meyers-Brigs Type Indicator likes a quiet space and prefers to work without interruptions. This learner probably prefers to work alone rather than in groups, and in a group situation probably offers personal opinions only if asked by others and may feel uncomfortable expressing opinions. The learner usually asks questions to clarify information and improve understanding rather than to understand the instructor's expectations and prefers to deal with thoughts and ideas rather than action and experience.

41. C: A behavioral objective in the affective domain at the characterization level (indicating integration of values) is: Following a series of class sessions about ethics and confidentiality, the learner will show consistent interest in respecting client's rights and protecting confidentiality. The affective (feeling) domain can be hard to measure, and evaluation is usually subjective based on inference; so the nurse educator must look for evidence of interest, commitment, and change in attitudes or behavior. Some use a Likert scale to help measure learner beliefs, attitudes, and values.

42. A: The three variables that the nurse educator should consider when choosing instructional materials are *learner, media*, and *task:*
Learner: Make selections that best fit the need of the audience, considering physical attributes, sensorimotor skills, literacy levels, cultural background, and learning styles.
Media: Exhibit flexibility in choosing a range of media (audiovisual, print, and demonstration) and avoid an over-reliance on print materials
Task: Identify learning domain (cognitive, affective, or psychomotor) and required behaviors as related to objectives.

43. B: Even though these learners are predominately visual and it's helpful to understand learners' learning styles, the nurse educator must avoid teaching primarily to one group but must focus on the needs of all learners, so the nurse educator should provide a wide variety of approaches that appeal to all types of learners: Provide written materials, graphs, charts, and videos; give explanations, answer questions; and provide materials for manipulation. Kinesthetic learners are often overlooked, especially when an instructor uses primarily a lecture format.

44. B: At a class level, the best method to assess a learner's cognitive knowledge base at the beginning of a course of study is to give a pretest because this highlights information that the learner already knows and serves to also alert the learner to important concepts that they need to focus on in the class. Pretests can help the nurse educator determine where the primary focus needs to be. Pretests are useful guides to learning, especially if the content of the pretest is covered and tested within a few days.

45. C: The best response to poor learner evaluations is to acknowledge the need to develop better strategies for teaching non-traditional learners. Younger learners are often used to group projects and feel comfortable working in groups, while older learners are often less used to this format and prefer to work independently. If not adequately prepared for group work, this can lead to conflict and lack of cooperation on the part of learners who feel their needs and preferences are being ignored.

46. D: The nurse educator should document observations of annoying behavior because behavior may worsen, and documentation establishes a record of the learner's behavior. The nurse educator can also use the documentation when meeting with the learner to discuss patterns of behavior that are of concern. Documentation is also useful if the nurse educator must refer the learner to someone else, such as a counselor, or if behavior worsens and disciplinary action is required. The nurse educator should avoid subjective comments and describe behavior in objective terms, including date, time, place, and witnesses.

47. A: Lecture and one-on-one instruction are almost exclusively directed at the cognitive domain of learning; this is the traditional focus of much of education where learners are passive recipients of knowledge and instructors are the providers. These methods remain two of the most common educational approaches, especially when one instructor needs to teach many learners; however, these approaches, especially lectures, do not engage the learner in activities that promote retention of information and they appeal to only some types of learners.

48. C: Willingham (2002) considered the "spacing effect" on learning and observed that there is a difference in retention depending on how information is learned. *Massed practice,* which refers to learning information all at once, such as during one cramming session, is less effective for retention than *distributed practice,* which

refers to learning information over a number of successive time periods. Studies indicate 67% better retention for distributed practice. Surprisingly, longer delays between practice result in more permanent retention.

49. D: Krathwol et al.'s (1964) levels of affective behavior include:
Receiving: Showing a willingness to focus on data and awareness of an idea.
Responding: Responding to experiences because required to initially and then because of personal will, leading to pleasure in new experiences.
Valuing: Accepting the value of a theory, idea, or event and showing commitment and preferences for some experiences.
Organization: Organizing and prioritizing values and incorporating new values into existing ones.
Characterization: Integrating values into a cohesive philosophy and demonstrating consistency in application of values.

50. B: Origination. Psychomotor skills are evaluated at seven levels:
Perception: Reads directions and observes processes.
Set: Exhibits readiness to carry out an action.
Guided response: Imitates and carries out actions with guidance.
Mechanism: Performs steps consistently with confidence and little hesitance.
Complex overt response: Performs steps automatically with no hesitance.
Adaptation: Adapts processes to fit the situation or individual needs.
Origination: Creates new motor acts or novel methods based on understanding and skills.

51. A: Return demonstration is the most appropriate method of evaluating psychomotor skills, such as administration of heparin. One purpose and goal—such as providing learners with knowledge necessary to administer heparin—may require a number of steps and a number of different evaluation methods. Identifying anatomic sites for injection may be assessed with a post-test. Drawing up the medication should also be assessed by return demonstration. Expressing concerns about the procedure is best evaluated through a question and answer session that allows learners to discuss their level of confidence regarding the procedure.

52. C: If a learner is failing to fulfill the terms of the learning contract, the nurse educator should discuss with the learner the problems he or she is having completing the contract. Simply asking "why" may seem accusative or threatening, and the reasons may be complex or even outside of the learner's control. In some cases, the contract may need to be renegotiated, while in other cases, the learner may need assistance with time management or other issues.

53. B: Regardless of how good the ideas for change are, a newly-hired novice educator who immediately begins making suggestions for change is likely to encounter a wall of resistance from those who are happy with the *status quo* and those who feel the nurse educator's suggestions are insulting to them. Additionally,

without knowing the organization well, the nurse educator may make suggestions that are not feasible. A wise course of action is to get to know the staff, observe, and participate before making suggestions.

54. D: Substantive due process is related to how the decision was made. The learner has a right to a fair and nondiscriminatory decision based on objective findings rather than subjective opinions. Procedural due process refers to the steps required when taking disciplinary action or expressing academic concerns, such as when a learner is failing. Procedural due process includes the right to a hearing, to notification of concerns, and the right to be heard (present a case).

55. C: The ability to communicate clearly may be a safety issue. In some cases, simply speaking more slowly and distinctly may improve communication, but accents are formed through time and habit and are difficult to change without help, even when learners are motivated. The best solution is to have the learning center (or appropriate department) develop accent reduction classes or modules to help learners identify their particular issues and focus on correcting those that cause the most difficulty with communication.

56. B: The best solution to prevent further plagiarism is to require all papers to be scanned through plagiarism detection tools. This is now common practice in many colleges and universities and not only helps to identify plagiarism but also helps the learners understand the importance of properly citing sources. Papers are submitted online and scanned automatically. Additionally, the instructors should keep copies of learners' papers, as plagiarism often involves turning in a paper written by someone else.

57. A: The person who is likely to be the most effective in helping to develop modifications for a learner with a BE amputation of the right arm is an occupational therapist, who can help to devise specific strategies to carry out procedures utilizing either the left hand alone or both extremities. The therapist should review the teaching plans to determine the types of activities the learner must perform in order to develop procedures and identify assistive devices that the learner can use.

58. D: The best course of action for a nurse educator who encounters an inebriated learner in class is to make an appointment with the learner and the program director (or other appropriate staff person) to discuss observations and substance abuse in an attempt to identify problems and to assist the learner. Since this is a classroom and not a clinical practice environment, the learner may be allowed to remain in class unless the learner is disruptive.

59. B: Bevis's (2000) illegitimate curricula is that which cannot be effectively graded or measured because it is hard to describe in behavioral terms. It includes qualities such as caring and compassion, which the nurse educator tries to engender in learners through discussions, observations, and role modeling; this curricula is

heavily influenced by the learners' perceptions, life influences, attitudes, values, and style. Illegitimate curricula also include the role of power and its use (or misuse). Other types of curricula include official, operational, hidden, and null.

60. B: While there is value in all of these approaches to disseminating information about a successful program, the best method is to submit an article about the model to a professional journal. Since professional journal articles are usually juried, submitting an article adds prestige and provides evidence of the quality of the program. Additionally, professional journals have the potential to reach a broader audience and more people in the profession. Before submitting an article for publication, the nurse educator should obtain writing guidelines for the target publication to ensure the article is written in the proper format.

61. A: Goodland's levels of curriculum planning:
Societal curriculum: Curriculum planned for specific populations of learners from outside the institution to standardize nursing education. Examples include guidelines prepared by the National League for Nursing.
Institutional curriculum: Curriculum prepared by the faculty for a group of learners. This includes global planning of the type of curricula and sequences of curricula.
Instructional curriculum: Curriculum developed by an individual instructor. This includes curriculum at the individual class level intended for the group of learners enrolled in the class.

62. C: Competent. Benner's stages (1984) of clinical competence and Dreyfus and Dreyfus's (1986) model of skill acquisition:
Novice: Not adaptable, rule governed, and little experience.
Advanced beginner: Some experience and able to develop some action principles.
Competent: Two to three years of experience and able to cope well with job requirements but still lacks flexibility and requires extra time for planning.
Proficient: Looks holistically at situations, guided by experience, and is adaptable.
Expert: Much experience and provides care intuitively rather than by rules. Understands and responds to needs easily.

63. A: Networking involves meeting and getting to know others in the profession, usually outside of the person's organization, so the best method is often to become active in professional organizations at the local, state, and national levels, as this exposes the person to active professionals with a wide range of experience. As a member of a professional organization, the person may also attend national conventions and join message boards developed by the organization.

64. D: According to Tyler, the four primary tasks to be completed when developing curriculum include:
Formulate educational objectives: Identify learner needs, society needs, expert advice, and philosophy and state inferred objectives; utilize a theory of learning,

screen the objectives against education psychology, and define and state the objectives clearly.
Select learning experiences: Make decisions about content and clinical experience.
Organize learning experiences: Relate learning experiences to provide continuity, sequence, and integration.
Evaluate curriculum: Review and revise.

65. C: Progressivism: Curriculum should focus on problem solving, critical thinking, and scientific research, and teachers should help learners learn how to learn rather than just teaching content. Essentialism: Curriculum should be the same but learners are allowed to learn at an individual pace. Reconstructionism: Curriculum should concentrate on the needs of society with focus on social and cultural issues. Existentialism: Curriculum varies widely but should focus on the right to choose and the human condition.

66. B: Many programs for clinical nurse specialists and nurse practitioners spend little time on learning and teaching theories or pedagogical methods, but knowledge of these is critical to effectiveness in teaching, so the new hires should undergo training in these areas. This training may help the new hires shift from an emphasis on sharing content to an emphasis on developing critical thinking skills. Mentoring, unassigned time, and orientation to the mission and philosophy of the program area are also important to assist the nurse in the transition from clinical practice to education.

67. A: While all of these are factors, the primary impetus for the rapid changes in curriculum that are currently occurring is changing technology. The curriculum must respond to changes in documentation (electronic health records), the need for evidence-based research (database searches), new surgical techniques (robotics, microsurgery), new equipment (monitors, alarms, smart phones, medication-dispensing carts), and new methods of content delivery (Internet, videos, simulators). Learners are much more technologically savvy than previous generations and expect to utilize technology.

68. B: The key issues facing higher education are affordability, access, and accountability. While at one time nursing education was free, the shift to a university/college model has markedly and steadily increased costs. Access to higher education is increasingly limited because of increased costs of education and living. Ethnic minorities are underrepresented. Accountability is another issue, as accreditation standards are more rigorous, and colleges/universities are more and more often required to report outcomes in terms of dropouts, completion of degrees, and job placement after graduation.

69. D: Environmental scanning involves monitoring and evaluating external information, usually through an extensive review of the literature, which may include the popular press, magazines, and journals in order to determine what

trends are evident in health care and education. Additionally, networking and attendance at conferences may help provide information. Projection uses current data to predict the future. Prediction uses laws, propositions, and theories to make future predictions. Conjecture uses subjective judgment (insight, knowledge) to make future predictions.

70. A: Delphi: This technique does not require face-to-face meeting. It uses a questionnaire that is sent out to members and then the results are compiled and new questionnaires are sent until a consensus is reached. Storyboarding: Members write ideas on adhesive paper and place them on a storyboard where they are grouped under various headings. Critical incident/role playing: Members portray critical interactions (learner and instructor) from different frameworks. Nominal group: Members write down ideas and then present them orally. After all present their ideas and discussion takes place, the members vote.

71. B: The focus of outcomes assessment as part of curricular design is primarily on learner learning—the knowledge the learner has actually gained and can demonstrate. Outcomes help the school of nursing to evaluate the quality of the nursing education and to identify areas of strength and areas of weakness that need revision. This curricular focus on outcomes is a shift from earlier models in which the focus was on course content and appropriate teaching strategies for that content.

72. C: The statements are written at three different levels requiring increasing levels of knowledge and skills:
Beginner: "Carries out assigned procedures for clients." The learner has basic skills and can read and understand a care plan.
Junior: "Modifies a plan of care based on client's needs and outcomes." The learner is able to exercise skills in decision-making.
Senior: "Develops a plan of care based on the client's goals and desired medical treatment." The learner has a good knowledge of disease and interventions and is able to exercise judgment in developing a care plan appropriate for client needs.

73. D: Active learning activities require learners to be engaged in a learning activity beyond simply listening, reading, watching, and taking notes (passive activities), which are common in the traditional lecture classroom. An example of an active learning activity is giving an oral presentation because this requires the learner to research, organize ideas, and make a presentation with each of these steps reinforcing acquisition of knowledge. Other examples of active learning activities include group projects, case study discussions, and simulation practice.

74. B: Learners should be able to meet the requirements for critical learning experiences in a variety of ways, so all should have opportunities to develop assessment skills, but they may develop these skills with different groups and ages of clients and in different situations. When designating learning experiences as

critical, faculty members should consider how those experiences can be achieved and avoid placing narrow constraints because learners are more likely to become proficient if they can practice these learning experiences in a number of different manners over time.

75. A: According to Halstead (2002), the essential teaching behaviors for those teaching Internet courses include providing rapid feedback and clearly stating evaluation criteria. The teacher for Internet classes must determine what types of interactions will occur synchronously and what types will occur asynchronously. Generally, most interactions are asynchronous, allowing learners to access the course at any hour, although the instructor may designate some synchronous office hours or hours for testing. Learning tends to be more learner-centered and interactions are Internet based (e-mails, chats, messaging).

76. D: Formative evaluations are used while something, such as a course, is in process in order to determine if it is effective or not. Reasons for doing formative evaluations include to determine the need for clarification of material, to evaluate effectiveness of learning activities, to assess learners' outcomes and abilities to apply learned skills, and to identify problems with the course. Summative evaluations are used at the conclusion of the course to evaluate final learner outcomes (grades, skills, knowledge), to determine the overall effectiveness of the learning activities, and to plan course revisions.

77. C: Cognitive development: The basic premise of this learning theory is that development proceeds in a sequential manner with uneven progress through several phases. Cognitive learning: The basic premise is that retention of learning is influenced by various conditions, which may modify cognitive structures. Behavioral: The basic premise is that all behavior is learned and can be modified through a system of rewards and punishment. Multiple intelligences: The basic premise is that learners have varying degrees of 8.5 different intelligences.

78. A: According to information-processing theories, episodic memory is the component of long-term memory that contains memories the person has of personal experiences because episodes of life are stored. Semantic memory contains interrelated ideas and meaningful information packaged into schemata. Procedural memory contains knowledge of specific skills and tasks. Information-processing theories are modeled after the computer and are described in terms of data processing. Memory chooses which data to process and converts it into meaningful information prior to storage in the sensory register, short-term memory, or long-term memory.

79. A: The mentor's first action when noting that the novice nurse educator has missed a deadline should be to remind the person that the deadline has passed. The mentor's job is to support and teach, not discipline or report to the director of the nursing program for minor problems. Reminding the person gives that person the

opportunity to ask for help or indicate why the deadline was missed. If the person does not respond to the reminder, then the mentor may need to provide more direct coaching as to the reason the course outline needs to be submitted in a timely manner.

80. D: While complaints serve some purpose, they are often less productive than taking positive action, such as running for a seat on the faculty senate in order to make changes. Working from the inside, the nurse educator will have better knowledge of the function of the body and the limitations of its authority. While faculty senates may advise and collaborate in decision-making, the faculty senate recommendations are not binding, and final decisions almost always rest with the administration.

81. C: *Creating an anticipatory set* involves creating an environment that promotes learner interest. The three elements of an anticipatory set are active participation, relevance to learners, and relevance to class. Planning learning experiences involves a number of other steps:
Determine learning outcomes: Should connect to overall curricular goals.
Create an anticipatory set: (see above)
Choose teaching/learning strategies: Should consider content, educational philosophy, and feasibility. Strategies should be varied.
Design closure for activity: May include summary, review, question and answer.
Design formative/summative evaluations.

82. D: Learners often find it hard to remain engaged in lectures, especially if the material is presented over long periods of time, so the best option is to break the lecture into two 20- to 25-minute lecture periods with 5 to 10 minutes of discussion after each period, depending on the amount of content that must be covered. The nurse educator can also keep learners engaged by asking occasional questions of the audience members and using audiovisual materials.

83. A: Collaboration is an essential element when the nurse educator is using adult learning principles to work with adult learners. The adult must be an active participant in establishing learning goals and determining their own learning experiences. While adults tend to be self-directed, not all adults feel comfortable applying this self-direction to education, so the nurse educator must provide guidance to allay the fear of failure that is also common among adults. The primary role of the nurse educator is that of facilitator.

84. B: Phenomenology: An inductive research method used to describe the human experience and how and why people experience events. Learners may learn techniques of open-ended questions to utilize with clients in order to gain knowledge of the clients' life experiences. Post-modern discourse: This method focuses on determining what is real and true, recognizing that truth is a process that changes over time. Feminist pedagogy: This focus is on emancipation, intellectual

growth, and empowerment of the female. Critical pedagogy: This method focuses on analysis of power and the relationships that occur within social structures.

85. C: Cheating is considered an administrative violation because it is prohibited in the code of ethics for the school. In the continuum of misconduct, annoying acts, such as refusing to cooperate or texting in class, are at one end of the spectrum, followed by administrative violations, with criminal conduct, such as hitting another class member, at the other end. All levels of misconduct may result in some type of disciplinary action, although annoying acts can often be dealt with on a one-to-one basis with the nurse educator and the learner.

86. B: The use of games in class is most appropriate for knowledge reinforcement and may be used to review concepts that learners have already studied. Because games are often fun for participants, they may increase retention and motivate learners to learn. However, some learners may be uncomfortable with games, and preparing or purchasing games may be time-consuming and/or expensive for the instructor. The nurse educator must allow the games to be learner-centered and should clearly explain the rules and then conduct a debriefing at the end of the game.

87. A: Role-playing can bring up situations or issues that feel threatening to participants, so if the role-playing gets out of hand or participants are responding inappropriately, the nurse educator should suspend the role-playing and suggest that the participants and group discuss what just occurred, what triggered the response, and how the situation might be handled in a clinical setting with clients, using the interaction as a learning experience rather than a problem.

88. C: Relative (curve) grading drops the top score to achieve an A down to help compensate for the questions that are ambiguous or too difficult. However, using a relative grading system with a straight 10% dividing the grades groups the grades that are far apart in points in some cases and gives different grades to scores that are close in points in others. The best solution is to utilize a relative grading system that groups scores close in points, taking into consideration that a very high or very low score may skew the results slightly.

89. D: The one-minute essay with an open-ended question is likely the best choice for a CAT to determine if learners are able to identify the most important issues. With multiple choice and true/false questionnaires, the nurse educator must provide information about the important issues, and the choices given may not reflect what the learners actually believe. Discussion periods may not involve all class members, and some learners may simply agree with others. The one-minute essay forces the learners to think and respond independently.

90. A: While there is value to all of these approaches to multicultural education, the most beneficial is likely to be guest speakers from different cultural groups

discussing cultural/health attitudes, especially if the speakers participate in question-and-answer sessions, because learners often have little or no contact with different cultural groups. Guest speakers may include individuals or groups of individuals and formats may vary somewhat, but the nurse educator should find guest speakers who would feel comfortable addressing a group of learners.

91. B: Learners who are used to passive roles in class often find the transition to becoming an active participant very intimidating, so the nurse educator should devise developmental strategies to help the learners learn to participate and to be less fearful. The best solution is not to switch to a lecture format but to develop structural small group exercises that require interaction because learners are likely to feel less intimidated by speaking in a small group of peers without the direct close supervision of the instructor.

92. D: The three criteria required for cultural competence include *knowledge, skills,* and *acceptance:*
Knowledge: Information about different cultures and ethnic groups. The nurse educator should make sure learners receive appropriate cultural information.
Skills: The ability to incorporate knowledge of different cultures and ethnic groups into nursing practice and plans of care as well as communicate effectively.
Attitudes: Exhibiting behavior that indicates positive attitudes toward others. Attitudes are almost impossible to evaluate objectively, and people can project an attitude that they don't feel, so actions and reactions are important.

93. A: Male learners need to acquire the same skills and undergo the same training as female learners although the nurse educator must acknowledge their concerns, the same concerns some female learners have in relation to caring for male clients. The most appropriate solution in this case is to have a discussion about the issue of inappropriate touching vs. medical examination, including methods to ensure that the client is not overly exposed and is comfortable and that the learner maintains a professional manner throughout the procedure.

94. C: Surveys of learners have indicated that the most important attributes of a clinical instructor are clinical skills and judgment. The learners depend on the clinical instructor to teach them, and the ability to share knowledge with learners is critical to the learners' development as nurses. Instructors must exhibit skills in three domains of teaching—instructional (utilizing effective strategies to facilitate acquisition of knowledge), interpersonal (establishing a trusting relationship with learners), and evaluative (demonstrating skills in judging performance).

95. B: The best response is "In retrospect, how would you respond differently?" This allows the learner to imagine a different scenario and discuss ways of responding that may help in future interactions. Because the learner brought the issue up in the conference, it's obvious that the learner is aware of not handling the situation well and should not be punished for honesty with criticism. Dismissing the issue with

"Everyone makes these kinds of mistakes" does not provide an opportunity for growth.

96. D: The first thing that a clinical nurse instructor must do before instituting nursing rounds (which takes the learners to the client's bedside for direct learning experiences) is to gain permission from the client, explaining the purpose of the rounds and the role the client will play (active or passive). Nursing rounds may be used for a variety of purposes, including demonstrations of wound care or equipment, interviews, observations, and discussions of client care issues.

97. B: With the paired model for clinical experience, the nurse educator pairs a learner with a staff nurse with whom the learner will work for a designated number of days while the remainder of the time will be in the traditional model. The faculty member continues to supervise, but the staff nurse plans the learning experience for the learner so the faculty member has more time to supervise other learners. This model works best if the staff member's caseload is not excessive.

98. A: The best method to assist learners to develop the skills needed to evaluate themselves effectively is to ask learners to evaluate their performances on a regular basis. The nurse educator may ask such questions as "How do you think you managed that client's care?" and "How do you feel about your performance?" This allows the learners to explore their feelings and shows them that the nurse educator is interested in their opinions and evaluations.

99. C: The most important factor when the nurse educator is selecting a preceptor to work with a particular learner in the clinical environment is that the preceptor communicates freely with the nurse educator. The nurse educator is ultimately responsible for supervision and evaluation, although the preceptor may participate in both formative and summative evaluations. The nurse educator should meet with the learner and the preceptor together to clarify goals and answer questions at the beginning of the learner-preceptor relationship.

100. D: With a clinical teaching partnership, the nurse educator at the school of nursing works together with a clinical nurse specialist who works at the facility where learners will do their clinical experience. The nurse educator schedules clinical experiences, but the clinical nurse specialist, working as an adjunct faculty member, performs clinical assignments and supervises the learners. This model ensures that the clinical experience is guided by someone with current knowledge and expertise and helps to alleviate the problems associated with a shortage of nursing educators.

101. B: Inserting an NG tube is the least likely skill to be available for learner practice. Alavi et al. (1991) classified skills into three categories according to how frequently the skill was utilized and how many opportunities were available to practice the skill:

Fundamental: Done daily with numerous clients, including assisting with mouth care, bathing, bed-making, utilizing body mechanics, and positioning clients.
General: Done frequently to assess clients' progress and condition, including administering IV therapy, catheterizing, and administering medications.
Specialized: Done less frequently and in more specialized circumstances, including suctioning tracheostomies and the oropharynx, performing eye irrigations, and inserting an NG tube.

102. A: Before implementing a simulation in the learning lab, the nurse educator should complete a checklist of required learner actions but should not prepare a guide specifying these actions because the point of simulations is for learners to utilize critical thinking skills. With practice, the nurse educator should be able to estimate the time needed for a simulation. To prepare for the simulation, the nurse educator should also ensure that all necessary equipment is available. In some cases, the nurse educator may have a role in the simulation, such as that of reporting nurse.

103. B: Four. The items analyzed should reflect the question:
Theories should be described.
Similarities should be explained.
Differences should be explained.
Personal theory should be developed.

The nurse educator must then describe what is required to earn an A, B, C, D, or F and how many points to apply for each of the four parts and for each grade level. A learner should be able to compare the rubric with the grade for the essay and understand how the instructor assigned the grade.

104. D: Observational learning effects occur when a learner observes behavior and the response to that behavior:
Disinhibition: Observing unacceptable behavior that incurs no consequences. The observer is more likely to also exhibit the same behavior.
Inhibition: Observing unacceptable behavior that incurs consequences. The observer is likely to avoid this behavior to avoid the same consequences.
Facilitation: Observing someone being rewarded for a particular behavior. This observer understands the value of the behavior and may want to imitate.
Imitation: Observing teaches a model of behavior that the observer imitates.

105. C: In order to ensure that learners encode learning into long-term memory, the nurse educator must include opportunities to review and rehearse lesson plans. It is not sufficient, for example, for a learner to practice a behavior only on one occasion. Rehearsing requires not just doing the behavior repeatedly, but also thinking about the behavior, such as applying a process to different situations or discussing various uses for a process. Learners should be encouraged to link current information to previous data.

106. C: When learners observe behavior from the nurse educator that models their own behavior, this observation coupled with past success helps them to believe they are capable and can be successful. These learners have high self-efficacy and confidence in their own abilities as well as motivation to do well. When determining the type of feedback to provide and the type of modeling to present, the nurse educator should keep in mind the importance of helping learners develop self-efficacy.

107. D: A key belief of the social reform perspective of teaching is that knowledge contains values and beliefs that must be examined and that this examination should occur before adopting knowledge. This perspective is based on the idea that the goal of education is to make substantive changes in the world, not just to transmit information. Learners are challenged to examine ideas that they take for granted and to look at things in new ways.

108. A: The best solution is to choose the alternative that allows the community some access to health education: diverting some funds to develop interactive Internet classes. While continuing the program with volunteers sounds like a good solution, depending solely on volunteers poses many problems; and often the majority of the work is done by a few people, resulting in resentment and ultimately burnout. The nurse educators may look for other sources of incomes, such as grants or donations, to maintain part of the program.

109. B: The option that may provide the best service to the community is for groups of learners to set up diabetic screening and information booths throughout the community in parks, churches, malls, and community centers. While volunteering at a free clinic may benefit the clinic, the clients are already coming for treatment, and the goal is to get more people into treatment. Handouts in the community often provide little benefit, especially in a community of immigrants in which many people may be illiterate and/or may fear authorities, and political leaders may have few solutions for the problem.

110. D: The best solution to provide additional practice for learners who have difficulty assessing heart and respiratory sounds is to provide an interactive Internet or CD-ROM program that provides examples to help learners identify abnormal cardiac or respiratory sounds. Learners often need repeated practice, so just listening to a client's lungs one time is probably not sufficient, and literature is of little help. While practicing listening with each other may help in learning where to place the stethoscope, most learners will have only normal cardiac and respiratory sounds.

111. C: When reviewing a videotape of role-playing with learners, the best response is one that encourages learners to make objective assessments of their own performance, allowing them to guide the discussion as much as possible as this

facilitates their development as nurses: "What do you see when you watch your interaction with the client?" While learners are often nervous when being videotaped, they are also often unaware of distracting habits, such as rubbing the hands together.

112. B: The best solution to arranging for a guest speaker when the speaker cannot be physically present is to utilize videoconferencing because this allows interaction between the guest speaker and the learners and keeps the learners more engaged than through other methods, such as showing a video, which are more passive. While the person may present essentially the same information in alternate formats, these formats do not allow for questions and answers, which are often critical to understanding.

113. A: If the nurse educator administers the same achievement test on two different occasions to the same group of learners and finds that the results are almost the same, the test has reliability. Some variation in scores is acceptable, but a learner who tests at 95% should test in that range (92 to 98%) on retesting and not have a score that is markedly different. Tests must be consistent in measuring attributes. Reliability results in tests that are reproducible and generalizable.

114. D: Evidence is required to validate an assessment instrument. This evidence may be based on a number of elements:
Content: Examine course content to determine if the test mirrors and adequately covers content.
Response process: Determine if the questions are measuring that which was intended.
Internal structure: Determine if there is a relationship between test scores and content.
Relation to other variables: Determine the relationship of the test score to external variables.
Testing consequences: Determine the benefits to testing.

115. C: Because the test does not appear to relate to the content studied in the class, the test appears to lack face validity, which results from how the test appears rather than from evidence of actual validity. In fact, many class tests and quizzes are prepared only with face validity and no real effort is made to determine factors such as validity and reliability; however, learners are more motivated to do well if they perceive that a test at least has face validity.

116. D: When developing test items, each item should be designed primarily to test mastery of learning outcomes and those behaviors that are specified in the learning outcomes developed for the course. Learners who have mastered the material should be able to demonstrate this on the test. Test items should be focused on important information and concepts rather than minor ones and should be designed

carefully so that the wording is not ambiguous and that the directions are clear and easy to understand.

117. B: Constructed-response test items are those that require subjective interpretations and opinions, such as completion, short answer, and essay questions. Completion and short answer questions are easy to write but scoring may be difficult because of different learner interpretations. Essay questions are also relatively easy to write but are very time-consuming to score. Selected-response test items are objective and the learner can only choose a response based on the item itself, but poorly constructed questions may skew results.

118. D: Email is a valuable means of communication between learner and instructor, but the nurse educator must learn to establish boundaries. The best solution is to set email "office hours" during which time the nurse educator will respond to learner emails. This time may be the same each day or may vary, but the learners should know the schedule. The nurse educator may find that a number of emails have similar concerns, and one answer could be directed at a group instead of all individual replies.

119. A: 12.

	Total items	Obj. 1-40%	Obj. 2-30%	Obj. 3-20%	Obj. 4-10%
Unit 1	60	24	18	12	6
Unit 2	40	16	12	6	4

The purpose of the blueprint is to link the test items to the course objectives in order to establish validity. The blueprint should be prepared before the nurse executive begins to actually write the test items. Utilizing a blueprint helps to ensure that the test covers the content in accordance to the importance of the information.

120. C: When developing a true/false quiz, the maximum number of repeats of the same answer (true or false) that the nurse educator should use in a sequence is four (TTTT or FFFF) because with longer sequences, learners tend to focus more on the repeats than the facts and assume that the instructor would not have so many repeats; thus, they may doubt their answers. Additionally, question length should be similar, and the nurse educator should avoid patterns, such as TTFFTTFF.

121. A: The most effective method of preventing cheating among learners is to assign seats different from usual seating, making sure that close friends and study partners are seated at a distance from each other and spacing the chairs as far apart as possible. Learners should have only the exam and the necessary writing utensil on the desk and all other items should be placed beneath the learners' seats, including cell phones and watches. The nurse educator should remain vigilant during the testing, watching the class instead of directing attention elsewhere.

122. A: Test A with a reliability coefficient of 1.0 has the most reliability. The range for the reliability coefficient is 0.0 to 1.0 with 0.0 indicating no reliability and 1.0 indicating perfect reliability (although it's unlikely that tests will achieve a perfect score). Nurse educators should utilize measures of reliability when developing tests. Simple reliability measures include testing/retesting and parallel form (giving the same person two different forms of the test and then correlating the scores), although most instructors now use computer software programs to assess reliability.

123. D: Since the immediate problem is that learners lack math and English skills, the best initial measure is the addition of a basic skills test, which should test math, reading, and writing skills. Some admission policies also require SAT scores, and many schools of nursing conduct personal interviews, depending on the type of school. Some state institutions require open admissions and are more restrictive on the types of measures that can be used to admit learners.

124. C: The nurse educator has taken a number of reasonable steps to help the learner to be successful—discussion, learning contract, and mentoring—but the learner has not shown adequate improvement in clinical experiences. Ultimately, the responsibility for a learner's success or failure lies with the learner. Some learners have no problem with retention of facts and do well on tests but cannot apply what they have learned. In this case, the nurse educator must fail the learner because the learner places clients at risk and has not met expected learner outcomes.

125. A: Reflective thinking requires the person to reflect on personal experience or attitudes. In this case, the nurse educator is reflecting on previous educational experience, evaluating it and assessing both the positive and negative aspects. Reflective thinking is a valuable tool to increase self-knowledge and may be done orally, but reflective thinking can also be done through journaling or artistic presentations (paintings, drawings). Learners are often asked to reflect on their clinical experiences as a tool to help them understand their own attitudes.

126. A: Using brief evaluations by learners at the end of each class session to determine what is effective and what is less effective in order to modify course content is an example of continuous quality improvement because the nurse educator is engaging in ongoing assessment in order to improve delivery of course content to learners. There is also an element of learner empowerment in utilizing the information obtained from learners to make substantive changes to content or delivery.

127. B: The nurse educator needs to discard or rewrite question 2. The P value, which should ideally be between 0.6 and 0.9, is low. Two of the distractors (C and D) have a positive PBI, while the correct answer (B), which should be >0.2, has a negative PBI. There may have been some confusion with the answer or guessing.

Note that while question 3 has a relatively low *P* value, the distractors all have negative PBI and the answer is positive, indicating the question is difficult but discrimination capability is high.

128. C: The best solution to low scores on one test, which may indicate a problem with the test, is to allow learners to complete an extra credit project in the area of their weakest test score (which for some learners may be a different test) if they wish, although it should not be required as it was not a requirement listed in the course syllabus. Discarding the exam may eliminate assessment of some course objectives and may affect the weighting of the content and objectives.

129. D: When a nursing program's NCLEX-RN pass rate has a sudden decline, the best beginning point for evaluating the reason for this decline is to review the NCLEX group-performance data, which compares the school's performance with national standards. NCLEX provides pass rate data to all participating programs, and these programs can also purchase curricular information, which can help to identify weaknesses in particular academic areas so that the program directors know where to focus attention.

130. A: Surveys of new graduates are best conducted six months to one year after graduation, as most graduates will be employed by that time and should have some idea as to whether they are well-prepared to perform as nurses. Surveys should also include employers, as they can evaluate whether graduates they have hired have had the necessary skills to perform in their roles. People may be more responsive to Internet surveys as they are usually faster to complete. Additionally, if the surveys include selected-response items, data may be tabulated by software programs.

131. C: The results of learner surveys and interviews should be presented to the program directors and board as group data only. Because the interviews were conducted by faculty members, these interviewers would be able to identify individual learner's surveys, so this is an issue of privacy. In some cases, learners who are particularly unhappy or completely satisfied with all aspects of the school may skew the final results, but these results are mitigated by including them with group data.

132. D: A primary component of Freire's (1970) theory of emancipatory education is reflection. Freire believed that reflection helped learners to think critically. Freire stressed the need for equality between instructor and learner and the importance of the instructor creating a culture of caring so that learners could assume responsibility for their own learning. He also believed that the traditional system of education supported society, which was oppressive and dehumanizing, and that education should combat this oppression.

133. B: The best method of developing a sample outline for a proposed course is to obtain course outlines from a number of different universities offering nursing

informatics classes and to look for similarities in content. Because a sample is not the same as the end-product, the nurse educator does not need to carry out extensive research or take a course in order to prepare this outline, but more extensive research will need to be done if the school of nursing decides to include such a course.

134. D: Observed communication skills between learner and client are not always representative of skills exercised when the clinical nurse educator is not present. Role playing may help learners develop strategies and surveys provide feedback, but one of the best methods may be to assign process recordings as a form of self-evaluation to encourage learners to think more about communication. Learners write down their exchanges with clients and then analyze their interactive communication, assessing both strengths and weaknesses.

135. A: The best approach is to meet with the learner regularly, providing formative evaluations and giving the learner remedial work, which may include a learning contract to help build skills. The nurse educator should ensure that the criteria for learner success is clearly stated and understood by the learner. The nurse educator should objectively document patterns of behavior that have placed the learner at risk. Depending on school policy, the learner may be placed on academic probation.

136. C: Under Chen's (1990) theory-driven program evaluation, normative evaluations are conducted to determine what the program wants to accomplish. Methods may include conducting surveys and utilizing focus groups. Normative evaluations may be used during program development as well as for program evaluation. The three activities related to normative evaluation include:
Goal revelation evaluation: Identify desired goals and outcomes for the program.
Goal priority consensus evaluation: Prioritize goals and outcomes according to the importance given by stakeholders.
Goal realizability evaluation: Assess consistency between program goals and activities.

137. D: Protection motivation (Prentice-Dunn and Rogers, 1986) explains changes in behavior in terms of a threat, which serves as a stimulus to develop coping appraisal and changes in behavior. This theory focuses on a response to fear or threats, motivating people to take protective measures based on how severe the threat is, the likelihood that the threatened event will occur, the ability of preventive behavior to mitigate the threat, and perceptions of self-efficacy (belief in one's ability to make changes).

138. C: According to research, in order to maintain a productive but positive working environment, a 3:1 ratio of compliments/recognition to criticism should be maintained. Ways in which to show positive recognition of co-workers include acknowledging when they have done something well or made a useful contribution: "That's a good idea." Another method is through an organizational reward system,

which may be simply acknowledging someone's contribution in time or effort. The more positive the interactions become, the more likely the group is to find solutions.

139. B: While all of these methods are worthwhile in support of legislation, the most effective method is to participate actively in professional organizations at the state level because they often have the resources and personnel to lobby more effectively than one individual. Because many members of professional organizations are not active, almost all state level organizations welcome participation and may assign members to committees according to their interests. Organizations may develop a number of strategies in support of the legislation.

140. D: The first step in facilitating change within an organization is to believe that change is possible and then make a reasoned consideration about where to begin and what steps to take to facilitate change. Once the nurse educator has made a plan, then the educator should take action. This usually involves doing research and convincing other members of the staff to support a proposal for change. Once change is initiated, the nurse educator must assess the results of change and develop a better understanding of the change process.

141. D: An increase in the NCLEX pass rate from 86% to 92% represents a substantial increase, and all of these responses are appropriate, but the best response is to immediately begin carrying out a thorough research of the program and the results to determine, if possible, what aspects of the changes in the program contributed to the increase. In some cases, isolated changes that might be applied across the board may have had a significant impact, but one cannot make assumptions about causation without evidence.

142. B: As soon as the nurse educator determines that there are errors in the manuscript, the nurse must notify the journal even though this means the article may be withdrawn from publication because to do otherwise would compromise the nurse educator's integrity as a scholar. If the nurse educator allowed the article to be published with errors and the mistakes were noted, it would call into question the content of the entire article, and the nurse educator would lose credibility.

143. C: The key factor in designing successful Web-based instruction is interactivity. Learners must be actively involved in the learning process while studying. Interactivity may take many forms. For example, learners may have to respond to questions or make decisions about proceeding with the materials. When designing Web-based instruction, it's important to consider the possibilities of the medium rather than simply converting traditional content, such as PowerPoint slides, into an Internet format. Learners should have opportunities, such as through chat rooms, to interact with other learners as well.

144. B: A nurse educator who is not in a management position but has been urged to take a leadership course will benefit because the nurse educator interacts with and

influences learners and professionals. Even though the nurse educator is not in management, the nurse educator is a leader for the learners enrolled in the program, for clients and staff members with whom the nurse educator interacts, and with peers in some cases, such as when serving as chairperson on committees. All nurse educators need leadership skills.

145. A: The nurturing perspective on teaching is based on the premise that learning requires both cognitive and affective processes and is impaired by anxiety and threats to self-esteem and that teaching requires the nurse educator to balance between challenging students and showing caring and support. According to this perspective, when a great deal is expected of a learner, then this must be matched by high levels of support. The goal is to build learner's self-confidence and sense of self-efficacy.

146. B: Context-based learning is a four-phase process that is a variation of problem-based learning.
Phase 1: Learners are presented with a situation that is examined and learning issues and information sources are identified. This discussion takes place in a tutorial group with 9 to 12 learners and a tutor.
Phase 2: Learners gather information and study independently or in a group, helping to develop self-directed learning skills. The tutor prompts learning through questioning.
Phase 3: Learners take the new information they have gathered and discuss it and apply it to the situation.
Phase 4: Learners reflect on the context and the learning process.

147. C: Everyone is responsible for identifying opportunities for improvement in healthcare because each group brings its own perceptions. Clients may view healthcare from the perception of their individual needs, while politicians must have a more practical view because they must consider the needs of the population as a whole as well as budgetary concerns. Administrators are concerned with the effectiveness of healthcare in terms of outcomes and costs, and educators are concerned with meeting client needs and learner acquisition of knowledge.

148. A: The statement that best describes the observation of the client in non-biased terms is "The client stayed in her room with the lights out and did not respond to questions." This statement only states the facts of the observation and does not assign a diagnosis ("depressed") or interpretation ("visibly upset"). "Non-responsive" can be interpreted in different ways (not answering, comatose), so it's a poor choice of wording. "Refused" and "rejected" both have negative connotations and should be avoided.

149. B: The four major components of the learning contract include *content*, *performance expectations*, *evaluation*, and *time frame*. Content includes the objective and activities, while the performance expectations outline exactly what is expected

of the learner and the method of evaluation for those expectations. The time frame is especially important. The learning contract should include the date the contract was negotiated, the total term of the contract, and the specific dates by which activities should be completed or objectives met.

150. C: According to Aggarwal, the *conservative principle* of curriculum development is that the educator must conserve that which is necessary for the current generation of learners while discarding that which is no longer required. Thus, during curriculum development, all elements of the curriculum should be considered, including past, present, and future needs, to determine their value in the past and their current value in order to determine if they should be included. This principle focuses on subject matter rather than specifically on learners.

Secret Key #1 - Time is Your Greatest Enemy

Pace Yourself

Wear a watch. At the beginning of the test, check the time (or start a chronometer on your watch to count the minutes), and check the time after every few questions to make sure you are "on schedule."

If you are forced to speed up, do it efficiently. Usually one or more answer choices can be eliminated without too much difficulty. Above all, don't panic. Don't speed up and just begin guessing at random choices. By pacing yourself, and continually monitoring your progress against your watch, you will always know exactly how far ahead or behind you are with your available time. If you find that you are one minute behind on the test, don't skip one question without spending any time on it, just to catch back up. Take 15 fewer seconds on the next four questions, and after four questions you'll have caught back up. Once you catch back up, you can continue working each problem at your normal pace.

Furthermore, don't dwell on the problems that you were rushed on. If a problem was taking up too much time and you made a hurried guess, it must be difficult. The difficult questions are the ones you are most likely to miss anyway, so it isn't a big loss. It is better to end with more time than you need than to run out of time.

Lastly, sometimes it is beneficial to slow down if you are constantly getting ahead of time. You are always more likely to catch a careless mistake by working more slowly than quickly, and among very high-scoring test takers (those who are likely to have lots of time left over), careless errors affect the score more than mastery of material.

Secret Key #2 - Guessing is not Guesswork

You probably know that guessing is a good idea - unlike other standardized tests, there is no penalty for getting a wrong answer. Even if you have no idea about a question, you still have a 20-25% chance of getting it right.

Most test takers do not understand the impact that proper guessing can have on their score. Unless you score extremely high, guessing will significantly contribute to your final score.

Monkeys Take the Test

What most test takers don't realize is that to insure that 20-25% chance, you have to guess randomly. If you put 20 monkeys in a room to take this test, assuming they answered once per question and behaved themselves, on average they would get 20-25% of the questions correct. Put 20 test takers in the room, and the average will be much lower among guessed questions. Why?

1. The test writers intentionally write deceptive answer choices that "look" right. A test taker has no idea about a question, so picks the "best looking" answer, which is often wrong. The monkey has no idea what looks good and what doesn't, so will consistently be lucky about 20-25% of the time.
2. Test takers will eliminate answer choices from the guessing pool based on a hunch or intuition. Simple but correct answers often get excluded, leaving a 0% chance of being correct. The monkey has no clue, and often gets lucky with the best choice.

This is why the process of elimination endorsed by most test courses is flawed and detrimental to your performance- test takers don't guess, they make an ignorant stab in the dark that is usually worse than random.

$5 Challenge

Let me introduce one of the most valuable ideas of this course- the $5 challenge:

You only mark your "best guess" if you are willing to bet $5 on it.
You only eliminate choices from guessing if you are willing to bet $5 on it.

Why $5? Five dollars is an amount of money that is small yet not insignificant, and can really add up fast (20 questions could cost you $100). Likewise, each answer choice on one question of the test will have a small impact on your overall score, but it can really add up to a lot of points in the end.

The process of elimination IS valuable. The following shows your chance of guessing it right:

If you eliminate wrong answer choices until only this many remain:	1	2	3
Chance of getting it correct:	100%	50%	33%

However, if you accidentally eliminate the right answer or go on a hunch for an incorrect answer, your chances drop dramatically: to 0%. By guessing among all the answer choices, you are GUARANTEED to have a shot at the right answer.

That's why the $5 test is so valuable- if you give up the advantage and safety of a pure guess, it had better be worth the risk.

What we still haven't covered is how to be sure that whatever guess you make is truly random. Here's the easiest way:

Always pick the first answer choice among those remaining.

Such a technique means that you have decided, **before you see a single test question**, exactly how you are going to guess- and since the order of choices tells you nothing about which one is correct, this guessing technique is perfectly random.

This section is not meant to scare you away from making educated guesses or eliminating choices- you just need to define when a choice is worth eliminating. The $5 test, along with a pre-defined random guessing strategy, is the best way to make sure you reap all of the benefits of guessing.

Secret Key #3 - Practice Smarter, Not Harder

Many test takers delay the test preparation process because they dread the awful amounts of practice time they think necessary to succeed on the test. We have refined an effective method that will take you only a fraction of the time.

There are a number of "obstacles" in your way to succeed. Among these are answering questions, finishing in time, and mastering test-taking strategies. All must be executed on the day of the test at peak performance, or your score will suffer. The test is a mental marathon that has a large impact on your future.

Just like a marathon runner, it is important to work your way up to the full challenge. So first you just worry about questions, and then time, and finally strategy:

Success Strategy

1. Find a good source for practice tests.
2. If you are willing to make a larger time investment, consider using more than one study guide- often the different approaches of multiple authors will help you "get" difficult concepts.
3. Take a practice test with no time constraints, with all study helps "open book." Take your time with questions and focus on applying strategies.
4. Take a practice test with time constraints, with all guides "open book."
5. Take a final practice test with no open material and time limits

If you have time to take more practice tests, just repeat step 5. By gradually exposing yourself to the full rigors of the test environment, you will condition your mind to the stress of test day and maximize your success.

Secret Key #4 - Prepare, Don't Procrastinate

Let me state an obvious fact: if you take the test three times, you will get three different scores. This is due to the way you feel on test day, the level of preparedness you have, and, despite the test writers' claims to the contrary, some tests WILL be easier for you than others.

Since your future depends so much on your score, you should maximize your chances of success. In order to maximize the likelihood of success, you've got to prepare in advance. This means taking practice tests and spending time learning the information and test taking strategies you will need to succeed.

Never take the test as a "practice" test, expecting that you can just take it again if you need to. Feel free to take sample tests on your own, but when you go to take the official test, be prepared, be focused, and do your best the first time!

Secret Key #5 - Test Yourself

Everyone knows that time is money. There is no need to spend too much of your time or too little of your time preparing for the test. You should only spend as much of your precious time preparing as is necessary for you to get the score you need.

Once you have taken a practice test under real conditions of time constraints, then you will know if you are ready for the test or not.

If you have scored extremely high the first time that you take the practice test, then there is not much point in spending countless hours studying. You are already there.

Benchmark your abilities by retaking practice tests and seeing how much you have improved. Once you score high enough to guarantee success, then you are ready.

If you have scored well below where you need, then knuckle down and begin studying in earnest. Check your improvement regularly through the use of practice tests under real conditions. Above all, don't worry, panic, or give up. The key is perseverance!

Then, when you go to take the test, remain confident and remember how well you did on the practice tests. If you can score high enough on a practice test, then you can do the same on the real thing.

General Strategies

The most important thing you can do is to ignore your fears and jump into the test immediately- do not be overwhelmed by any strange-sounding terms. You have to jump into the test like jumping into a pool- all at once is the easiest way.

Make Predictions

As you read and understand the question, try to guess what the answer will be. Remember that several of the answer choices are wrong, and once you begin reading them, your mind will immediately become cluttered with answer choices designed to throw you off. Your mind is typically the most focused immediately after you have read the question and digested its contents. If you can, try to predict what the correct answer will be. You may be surprised at what you can predict.

Quickly scan the choices and see if your prediction is in the listed answer choices. If it is, then you can be quite confident that you have the right answer. It still won't hurt to check the other answer choices, but most of the time, you've got it!

Answer the Question

It may seem obvious to only pick answer choices that answer the question, but the test writers can create some excellent answer choices that are wrong. Don't pick an answer just because it sounds right, or you believe it to be true. It MUST answer the question. Once you've made your selection, always go back and check it against the question and make sure that you didn't misread the question, and the answer choice does answer the question posed.

Benchmark

After you read the first answer choice, decide if you think it sounds correct or not. If it doesn't, move on to the next answer choice. If it does, mentally mark that answer choice. This doesn't mean that you've definitely selected it as your answer choice, it just means that it's the best you've seen thus far. Go ahead and read the next choice. If the next choice is worse than the one you've already selected, keep going to the next answer choice. If the next choice is better than the choice you've already selected, mentally mark the new answer choice as your best guess.

The first answer choice that you select becomes your standard. Every other answer choice must be benchmarked against that standard. That choice is correct until proven otherwise by another answer choice beating it out. Once you've decided that no other answer choice seems as good, do one final check to ensure that your answer choice answers the question posed.

Valid Information

Don't discount any of the information provided in the question. Every piece of information may be necessary to determine the correct answer. None of the information in the question is there to throw you off (while the answer choices will certainly have information to throw you off). If two seemingly unrelated topics are discussed, don't ignore either. You can be confident there is a relationship, or it wouldn't be included in the question, and you are probably going to have to determine what is that relationship to find the answer.

Avoid "Fact Traps"

Don't get distracted by a choice that is factually true. Your search is for the answer that answers the question. Stay focused and don't fall for an answer that is true but incorrect. Always go back to the question and make sure you're choosing an answer that actually answers the question and is not just a true statement. An answer can be factually correct, but it MUST answer the question asked. Additionally, two answers can both be seemingly correct, so be sure to read all of the answer choices, and make sure that you get the one that BEST answers the question.

Milk the Question

Some of the questions may throw you completely off. They might deal with a subject you have not been exposed to, or one that you haven't reviewed in years. While your lack of knowledge about the subject will be a hindrance, the question itself can give you many clues that will help you find the correct answer. Read the question carefully and look for clues. Watch particularly for adjectives and nouns describing difficult terms or words that you don't recognize. Regardless of if you completely understand a word or not, replacing it with a synonym either provided or one you more familiar with may help you to understand what the questions are asking. Rather than wracking your mind about specific detailed information concerning a difficult term or word, try to use mental substitutes that are easier to understand.

The Trap of Familiarity

Don't just choose a word because you recognize it. On difficult questions, you may not recognize a number of words in the answer choices. The test writers don't put "make-believe" words on the test; so don't think that just because you only recognize all the words in one answer choice means that answer choice must be correct. If you only recognize words in one answer choice, then focus on that one. Is it correct? Try your best to determine if it is correct. If it is, that is great, but if it doesn't, eliminate it. Each word and answer choice you eliminate increases your chances of getting the question correct, even if you then have to guess among the unfamiliar choices.

Eliminate Answers

Eliminate choices as soon as you realize they are wrong. But be careful! Make sure you consider all of the possible answer choices. Just because one appears right, doesn't mean that the next one won't be even better! The test writers will usually put more than one good answer choice for every question, so read all of them. Don't worry if you are stuck between two that seem right. By getting down to just two remaining possible choices, your odds are now 50/50. Rather than wasting too much time, play the odds. You are guessing, but guessing wisely, because you've been able to knock out some of the answer choices that you know are wrong. If you are eliminating choices and realize that the last answer choice you are left with is also obviously wrong, don't panic. Start over and consider each choice again. There may easily be something that you missed the first time and will realize on the second pass.

Tough Questions

If you are stumped on a problem or it appears too hard or too difficult, don't waste time. Move on! Remember though, if you can quickly check for obviously incorrect answer choices, your chances of guessing correctly are greatly improved. Before you completely give up, at least try to knock out a couple of possible answers. Eliminate what you can and then guess at the remaining answer choices before moving on.

Brainstorm

If you get stuck on a difficult question, spend a few seconds quickly brainstorming. Run through the complete list of possible answer choices. Look at each choice and ask yourself, "Could this answer the question satisfactorily?" Go through each answer choice and consider it independently of the other. By systematically going through all possibilities, you may find something that you would otherwise overlook. Remember that when you get stuck, it's important to try to keep moving.

Read Carefully

Understand the problem. Read the question and answer choices carefully. Don't miss the question because you misread the terms. You have plenty of time to read each question thoroughly and make sure you understand what is being asked. Yet a happy medium must be attained, so don't waste too much time. You must read carefully, but efficiently.

Face Value

When in doubt, use common sense. Always accept the situation in the problem at face value. Don't read too much into it. These problems will not require you to make huge leaps of logic. The test writers aren't trying to throw you off with a cheap trick. If you have to go beyond creativity and make a leap of logic in order to have an answer choice answer the question, then you should look at the other answer choices. Don't overcomplicate the problem by creating theoretical relationships or explanations that will warp time or space. These are normal problems rooted in reality. It's just that the applicable relationship or explanation may not be readily apparent and you have to figure things out. Use your common sense to interpret anything that isn't clear.

Prefixes

If you're having trouble with a word in the question or answer choices, try dissecting it. Take advantage of every clue that the word might include. Prefixes and suffixes can be a huge help. Usually they allow you to determine a basic meaning. Pre- means before, post- means after, pro - is positive, de- is negative. From these prefixes and suffixes, you can get an idea of the general meaning of the word and try to put it into context. Beware though of any traps. Just because con is the opposite of pro, doesn't necessarily mean congress is the opposite of progress!

Hedge Phrases

Watch out for critical "hedge" phrases, such as likely, may, can, will often, sometimes, often, almost, mostly, usually, generally, rarely, sometimes. Question writers insert these hedge phrases to cover every possibility. Often an answer choice will be wrong simply because it leaves no room for exception. Avoid answer choices that have definitive words like "exactly," and "always".

Switchback Words

Stay alert for "switchbacks". These are the words and phrases frequently used to alert you to shifts in thought. The most common switchback word is "but". Others include although, however, nevertheless, on the other hand, even though, while, in spite of, despite, regardless of.

New Information

Correct answer choices will rarely have completely new information included. Answer choices typically are straightforward reflections of the material asked about and will directly relate to the question. If a new piece of information is included in an answer choice that doesn't even seem to relate to the topic being asked about, then that answer choice is likely incorrect. All of the information needed to answer the question is usually provided for you, and so you should not have to make guesses that are unsupported or choose answer choices that require unknown information that cannot be reasoned on its own.

Time Management

On technical questions, don't get lost on the technical terms. Don't spend too much time on any one question. If you don't know what a term means, then since you don't have a dictionary, odds are you aren't going to get much further. You should immediately recognize terms as whether or not you know them. If you don't, work with the other clues that you have, the other answer choices and terms provided, but don't waste too much time trying to figure out a difficult term.

Contextual Clues

Look for contextual clues. An answer can be right but not correct. The contextual clues will help you find the answer that is most right and is correct. Understand the context in which a phrase or statement is made. This will help you make important distinctions.

Don't Panic

Panicking will not answer any questions for you. Therefore, it isn't helpful. When you first see the question, if your mind goes blank, take a deep breath. Force yourself to mechanically go through the steps of solving the problem and using the strategies you've learned.

Pace Yourself

Don't get clock fever. It's easy to be overwhelmed when you're looking at a page full of questions, your mind is full of random thoughts and feeling confused, and the clock is ticking down faster than you would like. Calm down and maintain the pace that you have set for yourself. As long as you are on track by monitoring your pace, you are guaranteed to have enough time for yourself. When you get to the last few minutes of the test, it may seem like you won't have enough time left, but if you only have as many questions as you should have left at that point, then you're right on track!

Answer Selection

The best way to pick an answer choice is to eliminate all of those that are wrong, until only one is left and confirm that is the correct answer. Sometimes though, an answer choice may immediately look right. Be careful! Take a second to make sure that the other choices are not equally obvious. Don't make a hasty mistake. There are only two times that you should stop before checking other answers. First is when you are positive that the answer choice you have selected is correct. Second is when time is almost out and you have to make a quick guess!

Check Your Work

Since you will probably not know every term listed and the answer to every question, it is important that you get credit for the ones that you do know. Don't miss any questions through careless mistakes. If at all possible, try to take a second to look back over your answer selection and make sure you've selected the correct answer choice and haven't made a costly careless mistake (such as marking an answer choice that you didn't mean to mark). This quick double check should more than pay for itself in caught mistakes for the time it costs.

Beware of Directly Quoted Answers

Sometimes an answer choice will repeat word for word a portion of the question or reference section. However, beware of such exact duplication – it may be a trap! More than likely, the correct choice will paraphrase or summarize a point, rather than being exactly the same wording.

Slang

Scientific sounding answers are better than slang ones. An answer choice that begins "To compare the outcomes..." is much more likely to be correct than one that begins "Because some people insisted..."

Extreme Statements

Avoid wild answers that throw out highly controversial ideas that are proclaimed as established fact. An answer choice that states the "process should be used in certain situations, if..." is much more likely to be correct than one that states the "process should be discontinued completely." The first is a calm rational statement and doesn't even make a definitive, uncompromising stance, using a hedge word "if" to provide wiggle room, whereas the second choice is a radical idea and far more extreme.

Answer Choice Families

When you have two or more answer choices that are direct opposites or parallels, one of them is usually the correct answer. For instance, if one answer choice states "x increases" and another answer choice states "x decreases" or "y increases," then those two or three answer choices are very similar in construction and fall into the same family of answer choices. A family of answer choices is when two or three answer choices are very similar in construction, and yet often have a directly opposite meaning. Usually the correct answer choice will be in that family of answer choices. The "odd man out" or answer choice that doesn't seem to fit the parallel construction of the other answer choices is more likely to be incorrect.

Additional Bonus Material

Due to our efforts to try to keep this book to a manageable length, we've created a link that will give you access to all of your additional bonus material.

Please visit http://www.mometrix.com/bonus948/nurseeducator to access the information.